WORKBOOK to Accompany ADVANCED SKILLS for HEALTH CARE PROVIDERS

WORKBOOK to Accompany

ADVANCED SKILLS for HEALTH CARE PROVIDERS

SECOND EDITION

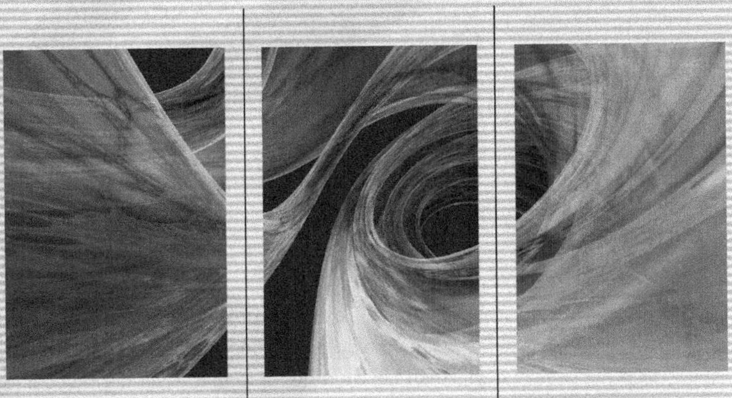

Barbara Acello, MS, RN

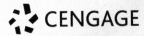

CENGAGE

Australia • Brazil • Canada • Mexico • Singapore • United Kingdom • United States

CENGAGE

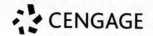

***Workbook to Accompany Advanced Skills for Health Care Providers*, Second Edition**
Barbara Acello

Vice President, Health Care Business Unit: William Brottmiller

Director of Learning Solutions: Matthew Kane

Managing Editor: Marah E. Bellegarde

Associate Acquisitions Editor: Matthew Seeley

Marketing Director: Jennifer McAvey

Marketing Coordinator: MicheleMcTighe

Technology Director: Laurie Davis

Production Director: CarolynMiller

Art and Design Specialist: Alexandros Vasilakos

Content Project Manager: Thomas Heffernan

Project Editor: Ruth Fisher

Library of Congress Control Number: 2005037322

ISBN-13: 978-1-4180-0135-3
ISBN-10: 1-4180-0135-X

Cengage
200 Pier 4 Boulevard
Boston, MA 02210
USA

Cengage is a leading provider of customized learning solutions with employees residing in nearly 40 different countries and sales in more than 125 countries around the world. Find your local representative at: **www.cengage.com.**

To learn more about Cengage platforms and services, register or access your online learning solution, or purchase materials for your course, visit **www.cengage.com.**

Printed at CLDPC, USA, 01-23

Contents

PART 3
Documentation, Documentation Exercises, and Forms 143

Preface

The content of your workbook follows a basic organizational pattern. To use it best, first review the key points from the corresponding textbook chapter. Do this review before proceeding to the activities. Each chapter has activities covering the vocabulary terms and other important content. These exercises will help you review, recall, reinforce, and apply the material from each chapter. Complete the workbook while the information is fresh in your mind. Students who complete activities such as these perform better, have more confidence in their abilities, and are more secure in the basic concepts than those who do not.

The development of critical thinking skills should be a lifelong quest for health care personnel. Critical thinking involves having knowledge and skills to process and generate information and beliefs, and the practice of using this information to guide your behavior and benefit the patients. Critical thinking involves actively and skillfully conceptualizing, applying, analyzing, synthesizing, and/or evaluating information gathered from, or generated by, observation, experience, reflection, reasoning, or communication, as a guide to belief and action (Scriven & Paul, 2003).

You will also receive many personal and professional benefits from critical thinking. The information in your textbook provides the basic foundation information you will need to think critically in your PCT role. The exercises and activities in this workbook help you learn to apply this information and become a critical thinker! You can make the best use of this information by:

- Reading and studying the related chapter in the text and doing the exercise at the end of that chapter.
- Observing and listening carefully to your instructor's explanations and demonstrations.
- Reviewing the chapter objectives at the beginning of each chapter when you begin the lesson. Review them a second time after completing all the activities to ensure that you have met them. Objectives map out the important points that you will learn in each chapter. Objectives are tools used to measure learning. They describe student behavior, performance, knowledge, and information gained as a result of the learning experience. Objectives are used to make judgments about learning. There are many types of objectives. Many of the objectives for the patient care technician are *behavioral objectives*. These describe behavior students must demonstrate or perform to show that learning took place. Because learning cannot be seen directly, the instructor must make inferences from evidence he or she can see and measure. Likewise, you should use the objectives to measure your own learning.
- Carefully studying the vocabulary words in each chapter so you understand their meanings and learn how to spell them. You will need to know these vocabulary words to understand chapter content and work in the health care field. These words are highlighted in your text and defined at their first use. The meanings are summarized in a glossary at the end of the textbook, which lists the terms and their meanings in alphabetical order for quick reference.
- Using the Key Points to quickly review and reinforce chapter content. The Key Points are a summary of important information presented in each chapter.
- Completing the activities in the workbook. Circle the numbers of any that you do not understand. Discuss these with your instructor the next day.

It is the author's sincere desire that this workbook will offer you support and assistance in learning and applying critical thinking. Becoming a PCT is a very special goal. Realize that to attain this goal, you must take many small steps. Each step you master takes you closer to your ultimate goal.

Barbara Acello

Acknowledgements

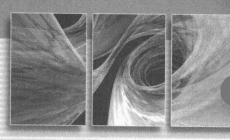

The author sincerely appreciates the kindness, support, and assistance of the following individuals:

- Terry Kotrla, MT (ASCP) BB, Austin Community College, Austin, TX, for the time and effort devoted to developing a wonderful Web page. Thank you so much for your responsiveness and prompt assistance in clarifying the laboratory reports!
- Laura Fowler, for her attention to detail, organization, and management of the numerous small details of manuscript preparation. Your willingness to give of yourself and your unfailing support made arduous tasks much easier!

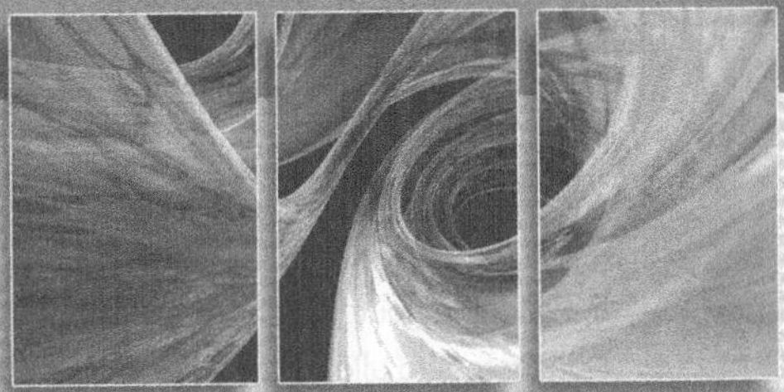

Tips on Studying Effectively

THE LEARNING PROCESS

Students may feel anxious about the learning process. Learning about health care is usually very different from other types of learning. Learning does not have to be a chore. In fact, it can be very pleasurable and rewarding if you have an open mind, a desire to succeed, and a willingness to follow some simple steps. You have already won half the battle by completing the nursing assistant program and enrolling in the PCT class. This shows that you are willing and ready to accomplish a commendable, real-life goal: becoming a PCT.

Steps to Learning

There are three main steps to learning:

- Active listening
- Effective studying
- Careful practice and application of the information

Students remember

- 10 percent of what they read
- 20 percent of what they hear
- 30 percent of what they see
- 50 percent of what they see and hear
- 70 percent of what they say
- 90 percent of what they see and do concurrently when performing a skill or doing homework, papers, or assignments

Active Listening

Listening actively is not easy, natural, or passive. It is, however, a skill that can be learned and mastered. In fact, mastering active listening will help you in many ways in both your career and your personal life. Good listeners are not born that way. They are made. In fact, they work hard to master this skill. Eventually, it becomes a part of them. The average listening efficacy in our culture is about 20 percent to 25 percent. This means that although you may hear (a passive action) all that is being said, you actually listen to and process about a fourth of the material. Effective listening requires a conscious effort on the part of the listener. The most neglected communication skill is listening.

An important part of your work involves listening to patients and coworkers. To master this skill, begin to listen actively to your instructor. Hearing but not processing the information puts you and the patients in jeopardy. Active listening requires listening with personal involvement. The three actions involved are

- hearing what is said (a passive voice)
- processing the information (active action)
- applying and using the information (active action)

Try to make your study area special. It does not have to be fancy. You should have enough light to see well, and a desk or table to work on. Have a supply of paper and pencils. Sharpen the pencils at the end of each study period and have paper ready for the next session. This may sound odd, but time is often wasted at the beginning of study sessions finding what you need. If these things are ready when you sit down, you can begin without distractions. Keep a medical dictionary and other study aids in your study area. When you get home, put your text and workbook there. Your work area is specifically for study. When you sit down, you will be physically and psychologically prepared to study.

Class Study. Now that you have your study area and schedule organized, think about how you can get the most from your class experience.

- Before class, get a good night's sleep and eat a balanced meal.
- Come prepared. Read the objectives and lesson before class. This familiarizes you with the focus of the lesson and vocabulary.

Steps to Planning

I. Block in the hours that are routine first (e.g., class hours, times to get children to school, clinical days)

II. Don't forget to allow travel time if needed

III. Plan responsibilities that must be met daily/weekly (e.g., food shopping, banking, church attendance, and other hour limitations)

IV. Plan daily study time

V. Plan regular recreation time

VI. Reevaluate plan after the first week and make necessary adjustments

		7 Day Planning Calendar						
Date	Hour	Mon	Tues	Wed	Thur	Fri	Sat	Sun
	6–7 am							
	7–8							
	8–9							
	9–10							
	10–11							
	11–12							
	12–1							
	1–2							
	2–3							
	3–4							
	4–5							
	5–6							
	6–7							
	7–8							
	8–9							
	9–10							
	10–11							
	11–12							

Figure 1 Write a weekly schedule, hour by hour. Analyze it to see how you are using your time. Block out a realistic time period for study. You deserve this time to invest in yourself, your future, and your career.

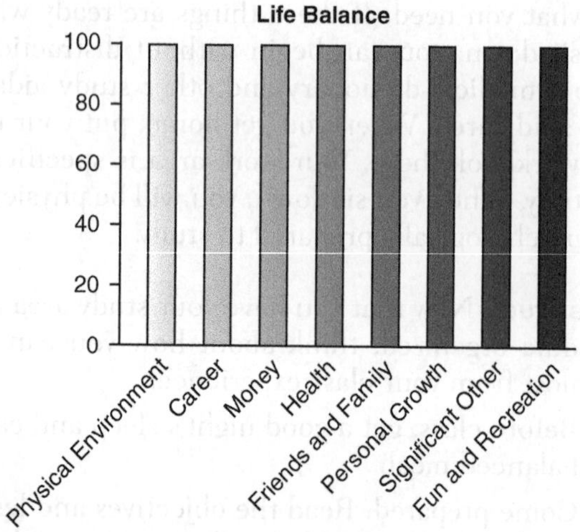

Figure 2A If your life is well balanced, each section takes an equal amount of time and energy.

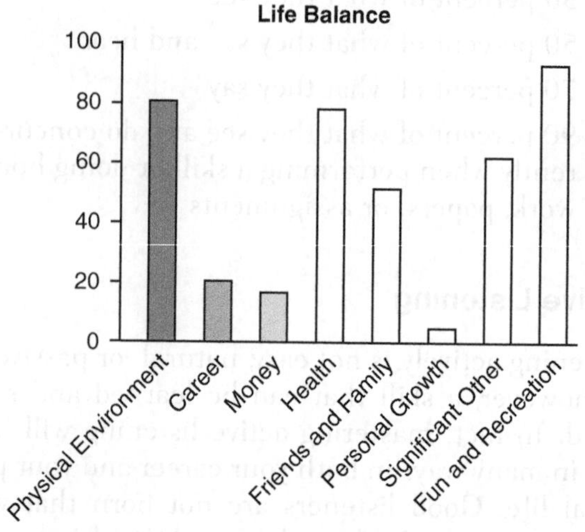

Figure 2B This shows a life that is not well balanced. If your life is out of balance, you have a bumpy road.

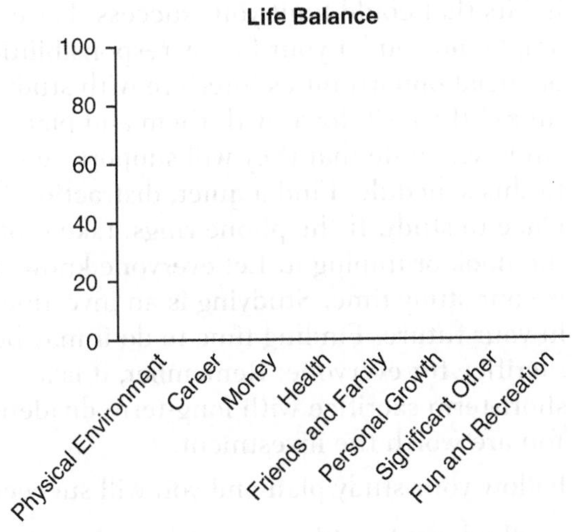

Figure 2C Use this chart to identify areas of your life that need balance. Draw a line showing the time and energy devoted to each area of your life.

- Come to class prepared, willing, and anxious to learn. Your success is affected by your attitude toward learning.
- Listen actively to what the instructor is saying. If your mind starts to wander, refocus immediately.
- Take notes on special points. Use these to study at home.
- Participate in class activities and discussions. These subjects have been selected because they relate to the lesson. You can learn much by listening to others' comments and by contributing comments of your own.
- Pay attention to teaching aids such as videos, transparencies, and posters. These provide a visual approach to the subject. You may wish to make notes of important points.
- Ask intelligent and pertinent questions. Make sure your questions are simple and focused on the topic. Jot down the answers for later study.
- Use models and charts, when available. Study them and see how they apply to the lesson.
- Carefully observe your instructor's demonstrations. Each state has acceptable methods of performing each procedure. Your instructor will inform you if the sequence in your state differs from the procedure listed in your text. Note state-specific changes in your book or skills checklists.
- Carefully practice skills and perform return demonstrations. Remember, these are real skills you will be using on patients in the clinical area.

After Class. After class is over, take a break. This will refresh you so you will be ready to settle down and study. You can gain the most from the experience by

- studying in your prepared study area. Everything will be ready and waiting for you if you followed the first part of the plan.
- reading over the lesson, beginning with the behavioral objectives.
- using a highlighter, pen, or pencil to mark important material.
- answering the questions at the end of the chapter. Check any that you found difficult or answered incorrectly by reviewing that section of the text.
- completing the related workbook lesson.
- reviewing the behavioral objectives at the beginning of the chapter. Ask yourself if you have met them. If not, go back and review.
- preparing the next day's lesson or assignment.
- using the medical dictionary to look up words that are not in the glossary. The dictionary will help you learn how to pronounce words you are unsure of.

Study Groups. Group learning involves using shared and learned information, values, resources, and ways of doing things. Groups become successful by combining all these factors. Each group and each individual is only as effective as the members are willing to embrace and respect differences within the group. Groups are most effective when members respect and encourage one another and have common goals and a commitment to learning the material. Studying with someone else who is trying to learn the material is very helpful and supportive, but there are some pitfalls you must avoid:

- Limit the number of people studying to no more than three; one other person is best.
- Stay focused on the subject. Do not talk about classmates or the day's social events.
- Come prepared for the study session. Have your work completed. Use the study session to reinforce your learning and develop a deeper understanding of the material.
- Ask each other questions about the material.

- Practice and use your active listening skills in your study group.
- Make a list of questions to ask the instructor.
- Limit the study session to a specific length of time.

Group members should:

- develop and share common goals.
- contribute to the group by sharing their understanding of the material, information, problems, questions, and solutions.
- respond to, and try to understand, others' questions, insights, and solutions.
- share their strengths and help others understand the source of those strengths.

Practice your procedure skills in your study group and have others critique you. Your instructor will evaluate your skills throughout your class. Others will watch you performing these skills in the clinical area. Practicing the skills in your study group will help you become comfortable with the procedures and confident in your ability to do them correctly. It will also help you overcome the nervousness and self-consciousness you feel when someone is watching you and evaluating your performance.

Each member empowers the others to speak and contribute. Members are accountable to one another. As a group member, you must learn to depend on others, but they also must be able to depend on you. The mutual respect, giving, taking, and sharing are the things that make a successful study group.

General Tips. The following are some general tips to help you study and master the material:

- Review the objectives when you begin to study. They are like a road map that will take you to your goal. Feel certain that each lesson you master is important in preparing your knowledge and skills. The workbook, textbook, and instructor materials have been carefully coordinated to meet the objectives. Read the objectives again when you have finished studying to verify that each has been met.
- Take responsibility for studying and take credit for your success. The instructor is your guide and the written materials are your tools. Using these things wisely is your responsibility. If you do so, you deserve credit for being successful!
- Take an honest look at yourself and your study habits. Take positive steps to avoid habits that could limit your success. For example, do you let your family responsibilities or social opportunities interfere with study times? If so, sit down with them and plan a study schedule that they will support. Adhere to this schedule. Find a quiet, distraction-free place to study. If the phone rings, take it off the hook or unplug it. Let everyone know this is your study time. Studying is an investment in your future. Finding time to do it may be a sacrifice for everyone. Remember, it is a short-term sacrifice with long-term dividends. You are worth the investment!
- Follow your study plan and you will succeed!

An excellent guide with many tips on learning to study, classroom participation, preparing for and taking tests, and learning in study groups is available online at http://www.studygs.net.

The MURDER Study System. "Study is nothing else but a possession of the mind" (Thomas Hobbes, 1651). Use the MURDER system to study each day:

Mood:

Set a positive mood for yourself to study in

Select the appropriate time, environment, and attitude

Understand:

Mark any information you do not understand in a particular unit

Keep a focus on one unit or a manageable group of exercises

Recall:

After studying the unit, stop and put what you have learned into your own words

Digest:

Go back to what you did not understand and reconsider the information

Contact external expert sources (e.g., other books or an instructor) if you still cannot understand it

Expand:

In this step, ask three kinds of questions concerning the studied material:

If I could speak to the author, what questions would I ask or what criticism would I offer?

How could I apply this material to what I am interested in?

How could I make this information interesting and understandable to other students?

Review:

Go over the material you have covered

Review what strategies helped you understand and/or retain information in the past and apply these to your current studies

Avoiding Procrastination. *Procrastination* is putting off or delaying something needlessly or unnecessarily. It is a bad habit for some people. To remedy procrastination, start with one project or lesson. If you are not sure how to reach your goal, discuss it with your instructor and ask for help or advice. Examine your attitude:

- Do you think this is just too difficult?
- Do you feel inadequate to meet the challenges of this class?
- Do you believe you cannot function without a lot of approval?
- Are you frustrated with the limitations of others?
- Do you expect nothing less of yourself and others than perfection?
- Are you convinced that disaster hinges on your actions?

These are all self-defeating, paralyzing, procrastination-producing attitudes and beliefs. Recognize them for what they are. Do not believe them and do not indulge in them! Replace them with positive, self-enhancing beliefs and attitudes. When negative thoughts sneak in, force them out with positive thinking, such as:

- I can do this. I am doing this.
- I am doing well with this. I have mastered ____.
- I can make the time for this and I can accomplish my goal.

The objective is to avoid wallowing in self-defeating thoughts and behavior by replacing them with positive thoughts and behavior. Over time, the positives will become a part of you, permanently replacing the negatives. Answer these questions:

- What do you want to do?
- What is the final objective of this project or lesson?
- What are the major steps to getting it done? (Answer this question in general. Do not get too detailed.)
- What have you done so far? (Remind yourself that you are part of the way there, even if it is just through thinking about it. Remember, the longest journey begins with the very first step!)
- Why do you want to do this?
- What is your greatest motivation for doing this? (Be honest. If your motivation is negative, reword it until it is written positively.)
- What positive results will you gain from achieving this goal? (Identifying these will help you discover hidden benefits that you may be avoiding. Dare to dream! List everything that stands in your way.)
- What is in your power to change?
- What outside resources do you need, if any? (Resources can include physical items, such as tools, money, time, people, and attitude.)
- What will happen if you do not progress?

Next, develop a plan.

- List major, realistic steps. Start small. A project is much easier when you begin with little steps. Add detail and complexity as you achieve and grow. Concentrate on small parts. Avoid thinking of it as an all-or-nothing affair.
- How much time will each step take? Develop a realistic schedule that will help you chart your progress.
- Identify specific study times that you will devote to yourself. This helps you develop a new habit of working, build a good work environment, and fend off distractions. (It is much easier to enjoy your project when distractions are set aside.)
- List how you will reward yourself at each milestone. Identify things that you will deny yourself until you reach the milestone.
- Schedule time for review. Ask a spouse, relative, or friend to help you stay motivated and monitor your progress.

Admit to

- false starts and mistakes as learning experiences. These can be as important as successes. Admitting to them gives meaning to experience.
- temptations. Do not deny they exist.
- emotions, including frustration when things do not go well

(Adapted from Hayes, John R. (1989). *The complete problem solver.* Hillsdale, NJ: Lawrence Erlbaum Publishers.)

Next,

- admit that you have had a problem, but also that you are doing something about it.
- see yourself succeeding.
- value your mistakes. Learn from them. Do not judge them and do not judge or devalue yourself!

If procrastination is a habit of yours, forget it. Focus on the tasks and project at hand, and build from there.

Practicing Carefully. Being responsible for the nursing care of others is a huge responsibility. To be successful you must learn to perform your skills safely, in an approved manner. There is a reason for each step of the skill, even if the reason is not apparent to you. Avoid taking shortcuts. Learn, study, practice, and apply your skills in the manner that you learn in class. To be successful as a PCT, you will need to commit the steps of these skills to memory so you can do them automatically. To do this, you must practice continually, in class and in your study group. Your instructor will plan skills laboratory and clinical activities to help you learn, develop, and master your skills. You have the responsibility to

- seek experience and skills you have been taught in the classroom and skills lab when you work in the clinical area. Inform your instructor or supervisor of skills you lack or those for which you need additional practice.
- practice your skills under supervision until you and your instructor believe you can perform them safely and correctly. Make certain your instructor evaluates your performance and checks off the skills on your checklist before you do them on patients without direct supervision.

KEY POINTS

Developing a few basic study habits can be important to a lifetime of learning. A few simple steps will make learning easier and will help ensure success in your future study endeavors.

- Be familiar with your text. This will save you time in finding information.
- Master the steps to learning.
- Practice becoming an active listener.
- Take notes for reference and study.
- Plan study times and practice in ways that promote learning.
- Work on creating balance in your life.
- Avoid procrastination.

ACTIVITIES

Vocabulary

Define the following terms in the spaces provided.

1. critical thinking ____________________
2. active listening ____________________
3. processing ____________________
4. procrastination ____________________
5. objectives ____________________

Completion

Complete the following statements by filling in the terms from the list provided.

10	active listening	imprint
20	carefully practicing and applying the information	key points
30	critical thinking	processing
50	distracts	
70	effective studying	
90		

6. The three basic steps to learning are ________________, ________________, and ________________.
7. Daydreaming ________________ you and interferes with your ability to listen actively.
8. The development of ________________ skills should be a lifelong quest for health care workers.
9. Students remember ________________ percent of what they read, ________________ percent of what they hear, ________________ percent of what they see, ________________ percent of what they see and hear, ________________ percent of what they say, and ________________ percent of what they see and do together when performing an activity.
10. The ________________ are a summary of important information presented in each chapter.
11. Taking notes is a good way to ________________ what you are processing.
12. ________________ involves making sense of new information in your brain.
13. As a PCT, you can and will make a difference in the lives of many others. Rearrange the letters to form a sentence in the lower grid, and think of how this relates to you, your class, and your chosen career.

A	G			H			4			D			E	L	A			
T	U	I	T	E	R	A	E	0	E	S		M	I	O	W	S	E	
B	O	T	F	L	A	V	N	D	T	H	E	S	P	C	E	T	R	
B	U	T	L	E	Y	F	L	I	0	0	E	L	I	E	M	E	F	R
											■					■		
					■				■									■
			■					■				■						■
		■				■					■						■	■

14. Follow the maze. Which path will you travel?

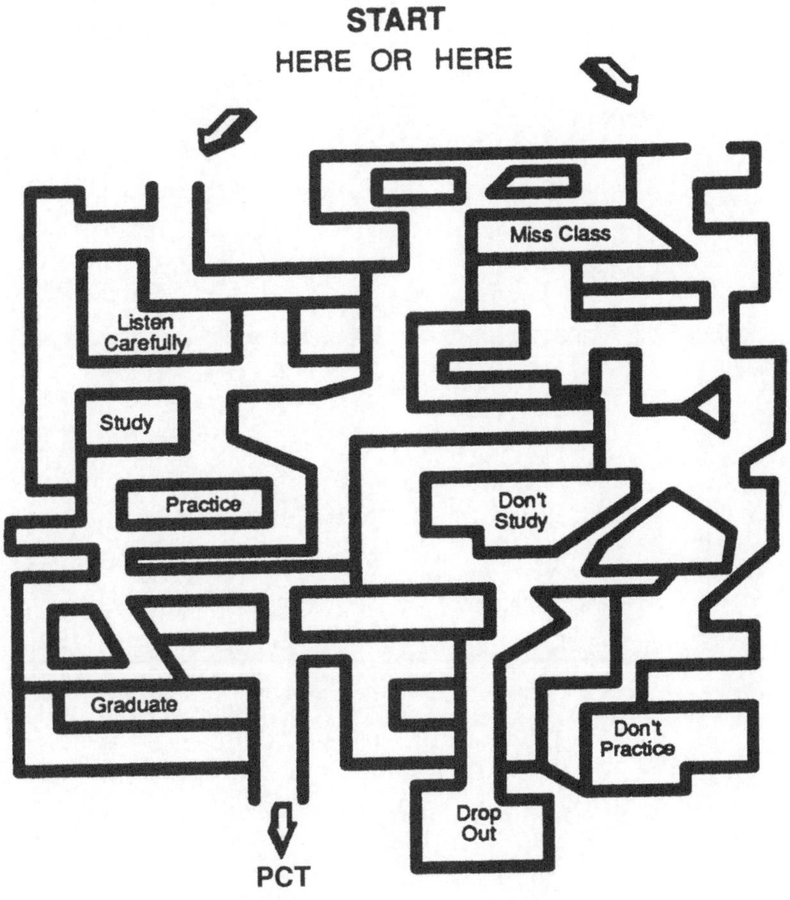

Figure 3 Follow the maze. Which path will you travel?

PART 1

Workbook Activities

CHAPTER 1

Health Care Delivery for the 21st Century

ACTIVITIES

Vocabulary Exercise

Define the following terms in the spaces provided.

1. barrier ______________________
2. benchmark ______________________
3. competent ______________________
4. critical thinking ______________________
5. delegate ______________________
6. denial ______________________
7. empathy ______________________
8. ethics ______________________
9. interdepartmental team ______________________
10. interdisciplinary team ______________________
11. intradepartmental team ______________________
12. intradisciplinary team ______________________
13. malpractice ______________________
14. multiskilling ______________________
15. negligence ______________________
16. nurse practice act ______________________
17. paraprofessionals ______________________
18. patient-focused care ______________________
19. professional boundaries ______________________
20. quality indicators ______________________
21. root cause analysis ______________________

22. sentinel event ______
23. standards of care ______
24. sympathy ______
25. tact ______
26. unlicensed assistive personnel ______
27. workplace redesign ______

Completion

Complete the table in the spaces provided by writing **PCT** *next to duties for which the patient care technician is responsible, and* **0** *(other) next to tasks for which other workers are responsible.*

Duty	PCT Responsibility?
28. Reporting unusual observations to the physician	______
29. Cooperating with quality assurance committee	______
30. Collecting specimens	______
31. Repairing electrical equipment	______
32. Delegating activities to PCTs	______
33. Starting and monitoring IV infusions	______
34. Using the computer	______
35. Passing medications to patients	______
36. Assisting patients with comfort, rest, and sleep needs	______
37. Assessing patients and developing care plans based on identified patient needs	______
38. Providing safe, age-appropriate care	______
39. Being empathetic and understanding	______
40. Providing perioperative care	______
41. Diagnosing illness	______
42. Applying the principles of medical asepsis in giving wound care	______

Complete the table in the spaces provided.

Age	Stage of Development	Developmental Tasks
43. Birth to 1 year	Infant	______
44. ______	1–3 years	Learns to differentiate self from other people
45. Preschool	______	Develops initiative and is able to plan and initiate tasks; recognizes self as a member of a family unit
46. School-age	______	Develops physical and mental ability; develops relationships with others
47. Adolescence	12–18 years	______

	Age	Stage of Development	Developmental Tasks
48.	________________	19–25 years	Establishes intimate relationships with a mate, spouse, significant other, or life partner
49.	Middle adulthood	26–50 years	________________
50.	Late adulthood	51–65 years	________________
51.	________________	65+ years	Does critical review of the events and circumstances of life; develops feelings of fulfillment, acceptance, and self-worth; copes with losses of friends and family; resolves remaining life conflicts and completes unfinished business

True/False

Circle T if the statement is true or F if it is false.

52. T F Sentinel events may also be called "near misses."
53. T F Intentionally unsafe acts result from criminal activity, purposefully unsafe behavior, alcohol or substance abuse, or patient abuse or neglect.
54. T F An adverse event may result from a commission or an omission.
55. T F Close calls are not given as much attention as adverse events that result in patient injury.
56. T F Patient care should be evaluated by the facility every two years to prepare for the accreditation survey.
57. T F Excessive noise delays healing, impairs immune function, and increases stress, heart rate, and blood pressure.
58. T F OSHA has set standards for noise levels in the workplace.
59. T F The purpose of patient-focused care is to bring patients to services.
60. T F Procedural errors and violations are the most common root causes of incidents.
61. T F The state nurse practice act does not affect PCT practice.
62. T F Health care workers must be competent in their responsibilities.
63. T F After a task has been delegated, only the person given the authority may perform the procedure.
64. T F In certain situations, delegating simple activities is inappropriate.
65. T F An RN may delegate the responsibility for patient assessment and care planning to an LPN/LVN or PCT if doing so is safe.
66. T F Identifying actual and potential health problems is strictly the physician's responsibility.
67. T F When you accept the responsibility from the RN for a delegated task, the RN is responsible for your actions.
68. T F The PCT may not refuse a delegated task.
69. T F Age is an important consideration in patient care.
70. T F The RN is the only employee who is responsible for teaching patients about safety.
71. T F Restorative nursing care is based on a belief in the dignity and worth of each person.
72. T F When applying the platinum rule, care for the patient as you think he or she wants to be treated.

Short Answer

Write the information in the space provided.

The principles of restorative nursing are:

73. ______________________________

74. ______________________________

75. ______________________________

76. ______________________________

77. ______________________________

78. Describe how critical thinking is used in root cause analysis.

____

____

____

Developing Greater Insight

Answer the following questions based on the situation described.

79. You are assigned to Mrs. Alexander, a confused patient. The critical pathway identifies her as a fall risk and notes that the two upper side rails should be up when she is in bed. The unit is busy and short of staff. Mrs. Alexander was in bed with the side rails down. You enter the patient's room and find Mrs. Alexander on the floor with signs and symptoms of a broken hip. She says, "A man hurt me." No male personnel are on duty. When you last checked the patient an hour ago, she was sitting in the armchair watching television. She had the call signal within reach. None of the personnel on duty will admit to putting this patient to bed, and you fear you will be blamed for the injury. The nurse instructs you to fill out an incident report. Mark the information below with an X if you will include it in your documentation.

________ unit very busy

________ patient was put to bed by another assistant with rails up

________ rails were not up when found

________ unknown how patient got into bed

________ patient was last seen up in chair an hour ago

________ patient confused

________ unit short of staff

________ patient says, "A man hurt me."

________ incident is the result of negligence

CHAPTER 2

Observation, Documentation, and Reporting to the RN

ACTIVITIES

Vocabulary Exercise

1.–15. Fill in the words in the puzzle using the clues and definitions provided.

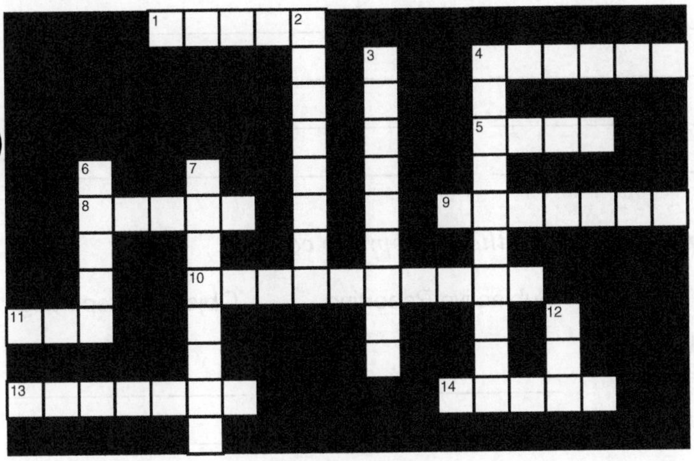

ACROSS

1. Things you can detect by seeing, feeling, hearing, or smelling.
4. You make observations about patients by using your _____.
5. _____ time is the best time for making patient observations.
8. Health Insurance Portability and Accountability Act.
9. Handwritten documentation in the chart must be _____.
10. Sudden, frequent, involuntary muscle contractions that impair function
11. _____-syncing involves linking a handheld computer to a full-size computer to update the information on both.
13. Patients' reactions to pain may be affected by _____.
14. The medical record is a _____ document.

DOWN

2. Things that the patient notices about his or her condition and tells you.
3. Factual observations.
4. Information the patient gives you that may or may not be true.
6. The _____ contains the patient's medical record.
7. Never give out your computer _____.
12. Personal digital assistant.

Differentiation

Differentiate between signs and symptoms by putting an X in the appropriate column.

Observation	Sign	Symptom
16. nausea		
17. vomiting		
18. diarrhea		
19. sore throat		
20. incontinence		
21. restlessness		
22. dizziness		
23. cold, clammy skin		
24. elevated blood pressure		
25. anxiety		
26. cough		
27. pain		
28. fever		
29. abdomen distended		
30. constipation		
31. rapid pulse		

Differentiate subjective from objective reporting by putting an X in the appropriate column.

Observation Reported to RN	Subjective Reporting	Objective Reporting
32. Patient made a face. She probably does not like her food.		
33. Patient found on floor. She states, "I slipped."		
34. Patient has a bruise on her hand and a skin tear on her elbow.		
35. Patient is rubbing her arm. It must hurt.		
36. Patient's urine has a foul odor. There are threads of mucus in the toilet.		
37. Patient is smiling. She is not having pain.		
38. Patient refused lunch. She probably was not hungry.		
39. Patient is sweating. Her skin is hot.		
40. Patient has been passing gas. She must be constipated.		
41. Patient has a fever and is shivering.		
42. Patient cannot find his room. His Alzheimer's must be worsening.		

Matching

Match the time with its equivalent in military (24-hour) time.

43. _____	3:13 p.m.	a. 2422	j. 1315
44. _____	12:43 a.m.	b. 1222	k. 2300
45. _____	9:10 p.m.	c. 2003	l. 0515
46. _____	12:22 p.m.	d. 0900	m. 1243
47. _____	5:15 a.m.	e. 1315	n. 1820
48. _____	10:38 a.m.	f. 0230	o. 1513
49. _____	8:03 p.m.	g. 0043	p. 1038
50. _____	11:25 a.m.	h. 1125	q. 2110
51. _____	6:20 p.m.	i. 1438	r. 1632
52. _____	9:00 a.m.		
53. _____	4:32 p.m.		
54. _____	2:30 a.m.		

Completion

Complete each statement as it relates to charting by selecting the proper word from the following list.

abbreviations	after	blank
color	entry	erase
facts	legibly	pencil
read	spell	title

55. Use the correct ____________ of ink.
56. Date and time each ____________.
57. Print or write ____________.
58. ____________ each word correctly.
59. Do not chart in ____________.
60. Do not use correction fluid or ____________ information.
61. Always chart ____________ giving care.
62. Leave no ____________ spaces.
63. Use only facility-approved ____________.
64. Chart the ____________, not your opinion.
65. ____________ what you have documented.
66. Sign each entry with your first initial, last name, and ____________.

True/False

Circle T if the statement is true or F if it is false.

67. T F Report subjective observations to the nurse promptly.
68. T F Changes that seem insignificant may indicate a problem.

69. T F Symptoms are things you identify with your senses.

70. T F Chart care that you know is supposed to be given, such as turning a patient every 2 hours, even if you did not have time to do it.

71. T F Use short, concise phrases in your charting.

72. T F If you forget to chart something, make a late entry in the record.

73. T F Begin setting your priorities when you listen to report at the beginning of the shift.

74. T F It is all right to read patients' charts to satisfy your curiosity.

75. T F The HIPAA regulations protect all individually identifiable health information in any form.

76. T F Computers used for documentation have audit trails that track the machine name, user, date, time, and exactly which medical records were accessed based on the user ID.

77. T F Documentation of information about patient elimination is not important.

78. T F Observation of the patient is a continuous process.

79. T F A common maxim in health care is, "If it is not charted, it was not done."

80. T F Hospital nursing units seldom use computers for routine documentation.

Developing Greater Insight

Answer question 81 based on the situation described.

81. Mrs. Maciejewski just returned to the unit following hip replacement surgery. The nurse informs you that this patient prefers to use the FACES pain scale. The nurse gave her pain medication at 3:15 p.m. At 4:30, you answer the patient's call signal. The patient is crying, points to the frowning face ("Hurts whole lot"), and tells you that her pain is number 4. You look at the patient's hip area, but do not see anything visibly wrong, then hand her the box of tissues.

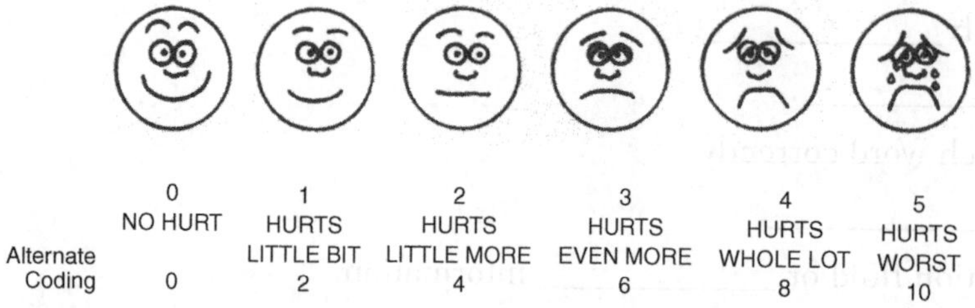

What does this pain level suggest? ______________________________

What action will you take first? ______________________________

What actions can you take to assist this patient? ______________________________

82. Nursing personnel diagnose and treat the human response to illness. Explain the main difference between nursing care and the care that physicians provide.

____

____

____

____

____

____

Answer questions 83–86 based on the scenario described.

Lynette has been running behind all day. Mr. Struck had an emergency in the morning, which caused her to get behind, and she could not get caught up. All her assigned patients were bathed and fed. At the end of the shift, Lynette completes her documentation and checks the flow sheets, which are complete. She documents intake and output, baths, and meal intake on her assigned patients. She started an IV on Mrs. Eager and ran it at a "keep vein open" rate. Because Mrs. Eager's IV was not started until after lunch, Lynette documents only limited intake and no output. She charts that she toileted Mrs. Eager every 2 hours, because she knows that this is the care she was supposed to provide. In fact, she did not take Mrs. Eager to the bathroom at all. The patient was not incontinent, so Lynette reasons that this omission was harmless. She did not inform the RN that the patient had not voided at all during Lynette's shift. After completing her documentation, Lynette leaves for the day.

Six hours after Lynette leaves the facility, Mrs. Eager is crying and complaining of severe abdominal pain. The RN assesses her and finds that the patient has a very distended abdomen. The nurse empties the patient's bladder with a catheter and obtains more than a quart of bloody, foul-smelling urine. She has to call the physician late at night to obtain orders for catheterization, laboratory work, and medication for this patient. The physician was asleep because he had an early morning surgery scheduled for Mr. Struck. The physician asks the RN about Mrs. Eager's elimination over the past 24 hours. The RN reviews the narrative documentation and flow sheets and informs the doctor that there were no abnormalities.

83. Was Lynette's documentation accurate and complete?

____

84. Could Lynette have managed things differently when she realized she could not get all her work done? If so, how? ____

85. Did Lynette's actions harm Mrs. Eager? Explain your answer.

____

____

____

____

86. Are there legal implications in this situation?

____

____

____

____

CHAPTER 3
Infection Control

ACTIVITIES

Vocabulary Exercise

1.–15. Fill in the words in the puzzle using the clues and definitions provided.

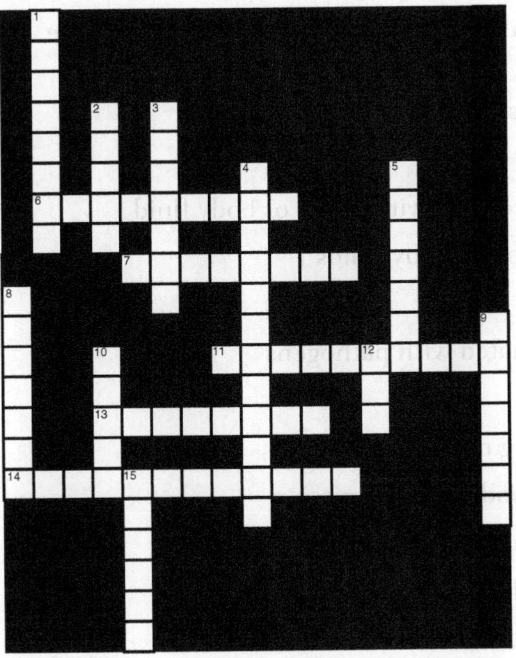

ACROSS

6. The place where the pathogen can grow.
7. A _____ pressure room must have at least 6 to 12 complete exchanges of air an hour.
11. Reverse or _____ isolation may be used for some patients who have diseases affecting the immune system.
13. Patients who have tuberculosis are placed in an _____ precautions room.
14. The mode of _____ is a description of the way the infection is spread.

DOWN

1. _____ precautions are used routinely in the care of all patients.
2. When caring for a patient who has an airborne infection, you should wear a _____-approved respirator.
3. A person who is able to spread an infection.
4. The use of biological agents for terrorist purposes.
5. A surgical mask must be worn when the PCT is within three feet of a patient in _____ precautions.
8. Patients who have infections of the skin and urine are placed in _____ precautions.
9. Insects, rodents, or small animals that spread infection.
10. An infection cannot spread if you break one link in the _____ of infection.
12. The government agency that makes recommendations to prevent the spread of disease.
15. Microscopic reproductive bodies that are very difficult to eliminate, and will multiply and continue to spread infection. They can survive in a dormant form until conditions are ideal for reproduction.

Matching

Match the terms and description.

16. _____ Tiny pathogens suspended in dust and moisture in the air that are inhaled by the susceptible host
17. _____ Insects or rodents that can carry disease
18. _____ Medications that eliminate pathogens from the body
19. _____ Place where a pathogen leaves the body
20. _____ A state of sickness or disease caused by pathogens in the body
21. _____ Spreading infection in food, water, or medications
22. _____ Describes what to do if you contact blood or body fluid at work
23. _____ Mucus and secretions containing a pathogen from oral, nasal, and respiratory secretions
24. _____ Type of isolation sometimes used to protect patients with diseases of the immune system
25. _____ Infectious diarrhea spread by spores
26. _____ Measures used when a patient has an infectious disease; prevents the spread of pathogens to others
27. _____ A bloodborne virus
28. _____ Microscopic reproductive bodies that survive in a dormant form for a long time and are very difficult to eliminate
29. _____ The use of biological agents for terrorist purposes
30. _____ Key to preventing foodborne infection
31. _____ Microbes that cause diseases to spread through contact with blood or body fluid
32. _____ Disposable items that are contaminated with blood or body fluids
33. _____ The way in which an infection is spread
34. _____ Touching objects, equipment, or dishes contaminated with pathogens
35. _____ Room used for airborne precautions
36. _____ May be safely used instead of handwashing during most routine care

a. Rotavirus
b. droplets
c. isolation
d. exposure control plan
e. indirect contact
f. spores
g. antibiotics
h. reverse
i. negative pressure
j. bloodborne pathogens
k. airborne
l. mode of transmission
m. portal of exit
n. biohazardous waste
o. common vehicle
p. proper temperature
q. alcohol-based hand cleaner
r. vectors
s. bioterrorism
t. infection
u. HCV

Short Answer

Write the information in the space provided.

37. Complete the chain of infection.

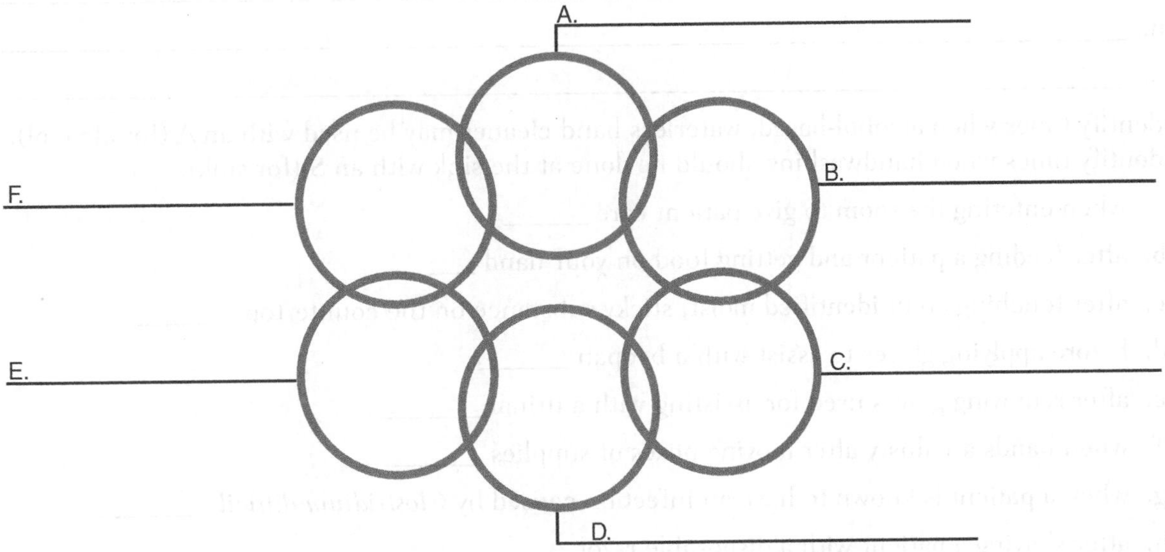

A. ______________________________

B. ______________________________

C. ______________________________

D. ______________________________

E. ______________________________

F. ______________________________

List at least five ways of breaking the chain of infection.

38. ______________________________

39. ______________________________

40. ______________________________

41. ______________________________

42. ______________________________

43. List at least 15 times when handwashing should be done.

a. ______________________________

b. ______________________________

c. ______________________________

d. ______________________________

e. ______________________________

f. ______________________________

g. ______________________________

h. ______________________________

i. ______________________________

j. ______
k. ______
l. ______
m. ______
n. ______
o. ______

44. Identify times when alcohol-based, waterless hand cleaner may be used with an *A* (for alcohol). Identify times when handwashing should be done at the sink with an *S* (for sink).
   a. when entering the room to give patient care ______
   b. after feeding a patient and getting food on your hand ______
   c. after touching an unidentified moist, sticky substance on the countertop ______
   d. before applying gloves to assist with a bedpan ______
   e. after removing gloves used for assisting with a urinal ______
   f. when hands are dusty after moving boxes of supplies ______
   g. when a patient is known to have an infection caused by *Clostridium difficile* ______
   h. after shaving a patient with a disposable razor ______
   i. before starting an IV ______
   j. after caring for a patient who has AIDS ______
   k. after caring for a patient in droplet precautions ______
   l. after caring for a patient who has a *Bacillus anthracis* skin infection ______
   m. before performing a sterile procedure ______
   n. after finishing a sterile procedure ______
   o. after caring for a patient suspected of having *Norovirus* diarrhea ______

45. List the order in which to apply gown, gloves, mask, and face shield.

______
______
______
______

46. List the order in which to remove gown, gloves, mask, and face shield.

______
______
______
______

47. Give five examples of fomites found in the health care facility.
   a. ______
   b. ______
   c. ______

d. ______________________________

e. ______________________________

True/False

Circle T if the statement is true or F if it is false.

48. T F It is not necessary to wear a mask when wearing a face shield or goggles.
49. T F Isolation categories are designed to interrupt the mode of transmission.
50. T F Artificial nails may be worn at work, but should not extend more than half an inch from the fingertips.
51. T F Many infections are spread on the hands.
52. T F Microbes may hide under rings worn on the fingers.
53. T F Tuberculosis is spread by the droplet method.
54. T F The susceptible host is the person who can become infected with a pathogen.
55. T F Rub waterless hand cleaners into the hands for at least 10 seconds.
56. T F Spores can survive in a dormant form for a prolonged period of time.
57. T F Alcohol-based hand cleaner will readily eliminate spores.
58. T F Protect yourself by wearing gloves for all routine patient care.
59. T F HIV is much more infectious than HCV.
60. T F Protective isolation protects personnel from contracting an infection.
61. T F Cutaneous anthrax cannot be transmitted from one person to another.
62. T F Items that have contacted blood or body fluids are biohazardous waste.
63. T F Food poisoning is an example of the common vehicle method of transmission.
64. T F Keep your fingertips up when washing your hands.
65. T F Change your gloves immediately before contacting mucous membranes and nonintact skin.
66. T F If you are splashed in the face with body fluids, wash the mucous membranes well with soap and water.
67. T F Standard precautions are not necessary when using transmission-based precautions.
68. T F Portable units can be used to create a negative pressure environment.
69. T F Facial hair will interfere with the seal of a respirator.

Identification

Identify the sign and indicate the type of precautions used.

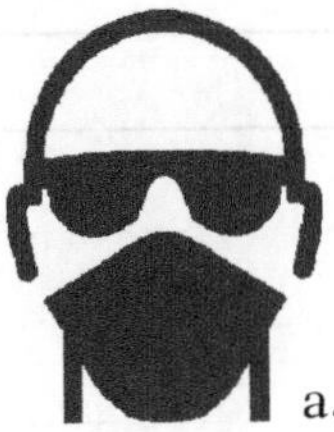

a.

b.

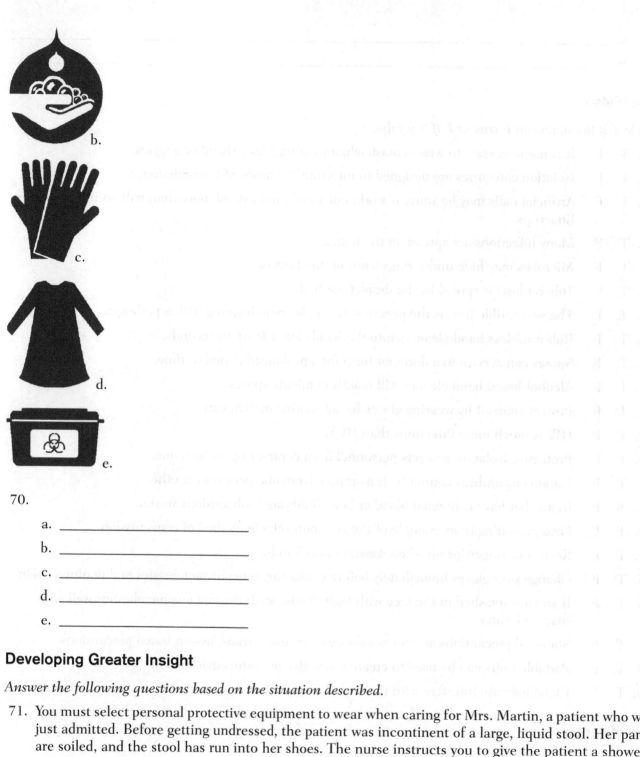

c.

d.

e.

70.

a. ______________________

b. ______________________

c. ______________________

d. ______________________

e. ______________________

Developing Greater Insight

Answer the following questions based on the situation described.

71. You must select personal protective equipment to wear when caring for Mrs. Martin, a patient who was just admitted. Before getting undressed, the patient was incontinent of a large, liquid stool. Her pants are soiled, and the stool has run into her shoes. The nurse instructs you to give the patient a shower.

    a. What protective equipment will you wear? ______________________

    b. Who are you protecting when you wear PPE? ______________________

    c. What will you do with the patient's soiled clothing? ______________________

    d. What will you use for handwashing before and after the procedure?

    Before: ______________________

    After: ______________________

Matching

Match each activity with the appropriate link in the chain of infection.

72. ________ Receiving antibiotics for an infection
73. ________ Disinfecting a bedpan
74. ________ Applying a dressing to a draining wound
75. ________ Not coming to work when you have a cold
76. ________ Applying a plastic bandage strip to a cut on your skin

a. protecting the portal of entry
b. protecting the portal of exit
c. protecting the susceptible host
d. controlling the causative agent
e. eliminating the reservoir

Identification

77. Identify what is wrong with each picture. State what should be done to correct the problem.

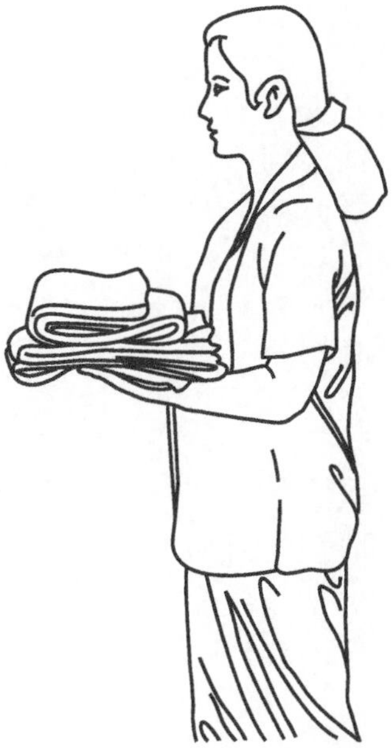

a. Error ____________________

b. Correction ____________________

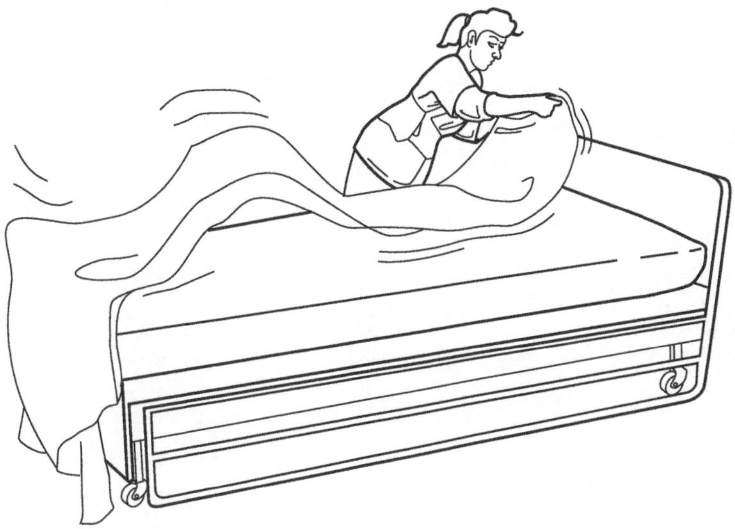

a. Error ____________________

b. Correction ____________________

78. What is wrong with the figure on the left? Correct it in the figure on the right. Use the empty bedside table to demonstrate the correction by locating the articles properly or writing in the words.

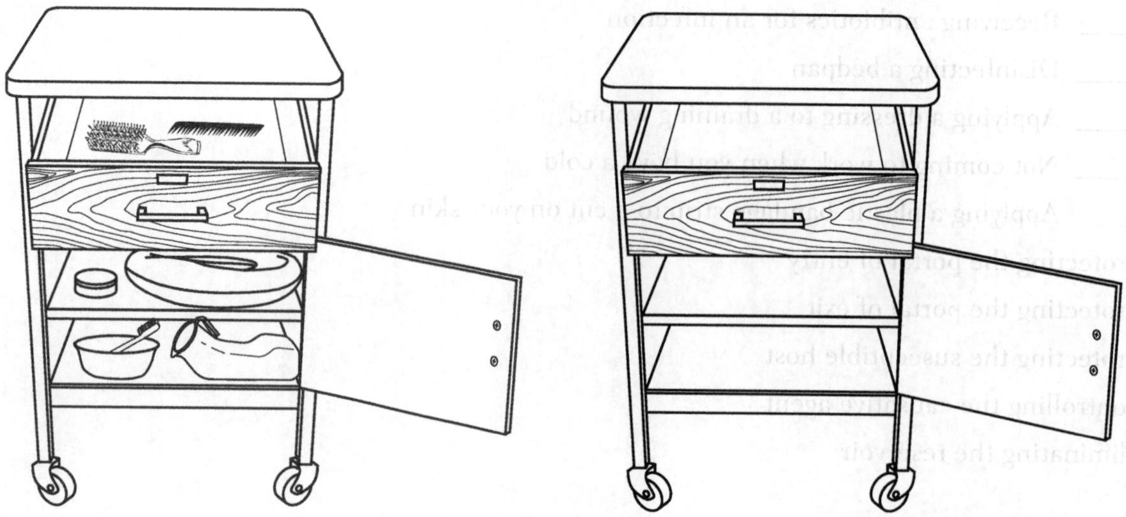

a. Error ________________________

b. Correction ________________________

CHAPTER 4
Surgical Asepsis

Vocabulary Exercise

Complete the puzzle by filling in the missing letters of words and key terms from this unit. Use the definitions to help you discover the words.

1.	_ _ S _ _ _	1. Farthest away from your body
2.	_ U _ _ _ _ _ _ _	2. Steam sterilizer
3.	_ R _ _ _ _ _	3. Covering for sterile packages
4.	G _ _ _ _ _	4. Worn on the hands
5.	_ _ _ _ I _ _ _	5. Closest to your body
6.	_ C _ _ _	6. Ten-minute wash of arms and hands
7.	_ A _ _	7. Covers the mucous membranes of nose and mouth
8.	_ L _ _ _ _ _	8. A type of waterless hand cleaner
9.	_ _ _ P _ _ _	9. Without microbes or contamination
10.	_ _ A _ _	10. Quick method of sterilization
11.	_ T _ _ _ _ _	11. Free from all microbes
12.	_ _ _ _ I _ _ _ _ _ _ _ _ _ _ _	12. Used during procedures to prevent contamination
13	_ _ _ _ E	13. Covers the sterile field
14.	_ N _ _ _ _ _ _	14. Describes procedure in which a puncture or incision is made into the skin or something is inserted into the body
15.	T _ _ _ _ _ _ _ _ _ _ _ _ _	15. Used to move items on a sterile field

Matching

Match the word on the right with the statements on the left.

16. _____	Sterile technique	a. steam
17. _____	Striped tape	b. proximal
18. _____	Used for surgical hand washing	c. expiration date
19. _____	Most common method of sterilization	d. surgical lubricant
20. _____	Document items sterilized	e. flash sterilization
21. _____	Contaminates sterile items	f. sterile item
22. _____	Date on sterile package	g. enzymatic cleaner
23. _____	First flap opened in sterile pack	h. distal
24. _____	Last flap opened in sterile pack	i. wet surface
25. _____	Work area for sterile procedures	j. sterile field
26. _____	Prevent contamination of sterile gloves	k. antiseptic soap
27. _____	Quick method of sterilizing instruments	l. log
28. _____	Commonly called "milk"	m. mask
29. _____	Removes protein substances	n. surgical asepsis
30. _____	Worn during some sterile procedures	o. keep hands above waist

Completion

Complete the following statements using the terms listed below.

avoid	discard	intact
border	drop	see
broken	dry	steam
contaminated	expiration date	surgical asepsis
corners	flash	wash hands

31. Sterile technique is used in procedures in which body cavities are entered or the skin is ____________.
32. Sterile technique is also called ____________ ____________.
33. Heat and ____________ in the autoclave kill all microbes.
34. Do not use a sterile package unless the outside wrapper is dry and ____________.
35. Instruct patients to ____________ touching sterile supplies, crossing over the sterile field, or talking or coughing over sterile articles.
36. Always ____________ ____________ before beginning a sterile procedure.
37. If a sterile item contacts an unsterile item, the sterile item is ____________.
38. Do not use a sterile package beyond the ____________ ____________.
39. ____________ sterile items onto the field from the sterile package.
40. Make sure you can ____________ your hands at all times when wearing sterile gloves.
41. When opening a sterile package, touch only the ____________ of the inner flaps.

42. Leave a one-inch ______________ around the outside edge of the sterile field.
43. When opening a sterile liquid, the seal should be ______________, and the container should not be broken or cracked.
44. ______________ disposable sterile supplies at the end of the procedure.
45. The surface on which you open a sterile package must be clean and ______________.
46. ______________ sterilization is a quick method used for sterilizing essential items, such as a one-of-a-kind instrument that was accidentally dropped during a sterile procedure.

Completion

Write the information in the space provided.

47. List at least 10 guidelines for sterile procedures
    a. ______________
    b. ______________
    c. ______________
    d. ______________
    e. ______________
    f. ______________
    g. ______________
    h. ______________
    i. ______________
    j. ______________
48. You must apply sterile gloves for a procedure. Place the steps to the procedure in the correct order by labeling them with numbers 1 through 12.

_____ Insert your right hand into the glove. Spread your fingers slightly, sliding them into the fingers of the glove.

_____ Check the glove package for sterility.

_____ Touch only sterile items with your sterile gloves. Avoid touching unsterile items.

_____ Insert your right hand under the cuff of the left glove and push the cuff up over your wrist.

_____ Insert the gloved fingers of your right hand under the cuff of the left glove.

_____ Slide your fingers into the left glove, adjusting the fingers of the gloves for comfort and fit.

_____ Wash your hands.

_____ Pick up the cuff of the right-hand glove using your left hand. Avoid touching the area below the cuff.

_____ Remove the inner package containing the gloves and place it on the inside of the outer package.

_____ Insert your left hand under the cuff of the right glove and push the cuff up over your wrist.

_____ Open the outer package by peeling the upper edges back with your thumbs.

_____ Open the inner package, handling it only by the corners on the outside.

Developing Greater Insight

Answer the following questions based on the situation described.

The RN asks you to set up a sterile field for a wound care procedure. The patient has been premedicated with a pain medication, and the procedure should be done within 15 minutes for maximum effectiveness of the pain medication. The nurse tells you she must obtain a culture and sensitivity test, then will cleanse a deep pressure ulcer, then pack the wound and apply a new dressing. She informs you that she needs a pair of size 7 gloves, a tray of sterile 4 × 4 gauze pads, two ABD pads, a package of Mesalt® ribbon, sterile applicators, sterile normal saline, wound cleanser, culturette, and a Kelly clamp.

49. How will you set up a sterile field for this procedure?

____

50. Are any items needed in addition to those listed in the scenario? If so, what?

____

51. The box of size 7 gloves is empty except for a one-pair package that is torn. What will you do?

____

52. You call central supply to obtain more gloves, and learn that no one will be available to bring gloves to your unit for at least 30 minutes. What will you do?

____

53. You have opened the tray of sterile 4 × 4 gauze pads and placed them on the sterile field. The patient sneezes. You do not know if she sneezed on the sterile items. What will you do?

____

CHAPTER 5
Wound Care

ACTIVITIES

Vocabulary Exercise

Find the words in the puzzle on page 26. If the word is part of a phrase, only the words in italics are hidden in the puzzle. Define each word or phrase in the space provided.

1. bandage ____________________
2. *continuous* sutures ____________________
3. cytotoxic ____________________
4. dressings ____________________
5. *granulation* tissue ____________________
6. *hydrocolloid* dressing ____________________
7. *hypoallergenic* tape ____________________
8. *interrupted* sutures ____________________
9. *localized* infection ____________________
10. *Montgomery* straps ____________________
11. *necrotic* tissue ____________________
12. *systemic* infection ____________________
13. *transparent* film ____________________

g	r	a	n	u	l	a	t	i	o	n	g	d	h
c	d	e	t	p	u	r	r	e	t	n	i	y	M
o	k	h	c	i	t	o	r	c	e	n	p	l	o
n	s	p	y	k	h	j	a	c	n	o	k	o	n
t	g	e	z	d	k	y	r	x	a	s	d	c	t
i	n	g	b	o	r	t	r	l	j	o	q	a	g
n	i	a	w	t	b	o	l	k	w	p	d	l	o
u	s	d	c	f	g	e	c	d	g	f	r	i	m
o	s	n	r	p	r	s	h	o	w	s	s	z	e
u	e	a	s	g	p	v	u	d	l	s	l	e	r
s	r	b	e	h	v	z	l	l	h	l	l	d	y
x	d	n	c	i	m	e	t	s	y	s	o	v	w
d	i	n	c	i	x	o	t	o	t	y	c	i	j
c	t	r	a	n	s	p	a	r	e	n	t	n	d

Completion

Complete the table in the spaces provided.

14. Stage ___ Partial-thickness skin loss involving epidermis, dermis, or both. The ulcer is superficial and presents clinically as an abrasion, blister, or shallow crater.

15. Stage IV ______________________________

16. Stage ___ Full-thickness skin loss involving damage to or necrosis of subcutaneous tissue that may extend down to, but not through, underlying fascia. The ulcer presents clinically as a deep crater with or without undermining of adjacent tissue.

17. Stage ___ Nonblanchable erythema of intact skin, the heralding lesion of skin ulceration. In individuals with darker skin, discoloration of the skin, warmth, edema, induration, or hardness may also be indicators.

Anatomy Review

Name the areas indicated in the figure by writing their names in the spaces provided.

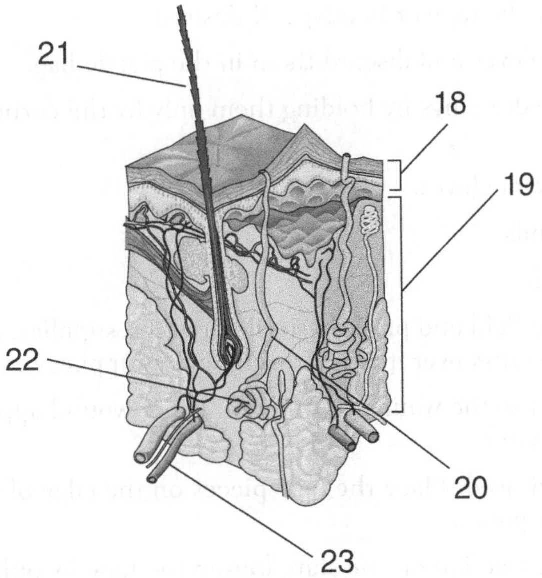

18. ______________________
19. ______________________
20. ______________________
21. ______________________
22. ______________________
23. ______________________

Write the information in the spaces provided.

24. List the 7 rights for dressing changes.

    a. ______________________
    b. ______________________
    c. ______________________
    d. ______________________
    e. ______________________
    f. ______________________
    g. ______________________

25. You must change a sterile dressing. Place the steps to the procedure in the correct order by labeling them with letters B through K. A and L have been completed for you.

A. Wash your hands.

_____ Tape the dressing securely in place, or cover it with a bandage. You may remove your gloves to apply the tape or bandage, if desired.

_____ Remove your gloves and discard them in the plastic bag.

_____ Pick up sterile dressings by holding them only by the corners. Center them over the wound.

_____ Apply clean exam gloves.

_____ Wash your hands.

_____ Apply sterile gloves.

_____ Set up a sterile field and prepare sterile dressing supplies. Arrange the field so that you do not have to cross over it when reaching for supplies.

_____ Cleanse and rinse the wound as ordered. If the wound appears abnormal or infected, notify your supervisor.

_____ Cut the tape, if used. Place the tape pieces on the edge of the overbed table, if permitted by your facility policy.

_____ Holding gentle traction on the skin, loosen the tape by pulling the ends toward the wound, and remove the dressing. Discard the dressing in the plastic bag.

L. Wash your hands.

True/False

Circle T if the statement is true or F if it is false.

26. T F Head lice hop, jump, fly, and crawl quickly from person to person.

27. T F Your bandage scissors are a potential source of cross-contamination.

28. T F Nits look like dandruff, and are easily brushed off.

29. T F Discard empty plastic catheter and dressing trays, and plastic bottles, in the biohazardous waste.

30. T F Head lice are tiny brown insects that are attracted to light.

31. T F You should never take the unit's treatment cart into a patient's room.

32. T F Liquid wound cleansers, such as normal saline, should be dated when opened, and discarded within 24 hours to 7 days, according to facility policy.

33. T F Nursing is an art and a science.

34. T F Wet-to-dry dressings are a dated method of treatment; other, less traumatic methods are more commonly used for debriding wounds.

35. T F An infected wound will not heal.

36. T F Transparent dressings are used to prevent the spread of infection from deep, infected, draining ulcers.

37. T F Transparent dressings may be used as a cover dressing instead of tape over a gauze dressing.

38. T F Transparent dressings promote a moist environment, which enhances and promotes healing.

39. T F A transparent film marked "for IV use" may be used to cover a small pressure ulcer.

40. T F The skin is the largest organ of the body.

41. T F A surgical drain is a potential portal of entry.

42. T F Patients should not shower with a transparent film dressing in place.

43. T F Use clean technique for providing pin care.

44. T F Systemic factors affecting wound healing are age, nutritional status, body build, presence or absence of chronic disease, circulatory problems, weakened immune system, and radiation therapy.

45. T F Necrotic tissue must be removed for proper wound healing.

Completion

Complete the following statements by filling in the terms from the list provided.

bandage scissors	granulation	separately
biohazardous	infection	standard precautions
clean	integrity	sterile
clean items	intravenous catheter	tissue
contaminate	moist	transparent film
dressings	once	up
environment	outward	
gently	room temperature	

46. When skin ____________ is disrupted, the patient is at high risk of infection.

47. Avoid contaminating the patient or the ____________ with your used gloves.

48. The overbed table is used only for ____________ ____________.

49. If the patient has multiple wounds, you should care for each wound ____________.

50. Wash your ____________ ____________ well with soap and water, then dry them after each use.

51. Position your plastic bags or other trash receptacle in an area that will not ____________ clean supplies.

52. Items that have contacted blood, body fluids, nonintact skin, mucous membranes, secretions, or excretions are considered ____________ waste.

53. Products such as peroxide and other solutions are not recommended for care of open wounds, such as pressure ulcers, because they destroy ____________ ____________.

54. Always place the lid or cap to a bottle with the sterile, top, inner side facing ____________ to prevent contamination.

55. Handle elderly patients very ____________ to avoid accidental injury to the skin.

56. If a wound irrigation solution is cold, let it stand until it reaches ____________ ____________.

57. Use an 18- or 19-gauge ____________ ____________ attached to a syringe to irrigate small cavities.

58. ____________ ____________ dressings are changed every 3 to 7 days.

59. Wounds heal best, and are less painful, in a ____________ environment.

60. When cleansing a wound, work ____________ from the clean area to less clean areas.

61. When cleansing a wound, use each gauze or swab ____________, then discard it.

62. A binder may be used to hold ____________, in place.

63. Any break in the skin increases the risk of ____________.

64. Always apply the principles of ______________ ______________ when caring for wounds.

65. Always use ______________ dressings to cover burns, surgical sites, and deep or extensive wounds.

66. ______________ technique is used when caring for superficial pressure ulcers and other minor wounds.

Developing Greater Insight

Answer the following questions based on the situation described.

Eric Rabb is a retired, 62-year-old, light-complected, African-American patient who was recently admitted with a diagnosis of venous stasis ulcers. He is 6 feet, 3 inches tall and weighs 252 pounds. He has a history of healed leg ulcers. At this time, he has painful ulcers on both lower legs. For the past two years, the wounds have been treated by his wife at home with daily gauze dressings and elastic wraps. The physician had ordered compression stockings in the past, but the patient seldom wore them. He said they were "too difficult for his wife to put on." When you remove the elastic wraps, you notice that the skin on the patient's lower legs is edematous, weeping, and an abnormal blue-brown color.

67. Based on your initial observations, what will you document about this patient? Write a short observational admission note.

____

____

____

____

____

Mr. Rabb was admitted to your hospital subacute unit for wound care and edema control. Severe bilateral lower leg edema made it difficult for him to walk and the painful, draining wound reduced his overall quality of life. The gauze dressings adhered to the wound bed, and the patient grimaced with pain when they were removed. The RN instructed you to measure the wound, and you found that the right-leg ulcer had an irregular shape, was 3.5 centimeters in diameter, and 1 centimeter in depth, with heavy, serous, and bloody drainage. The left-leg ulcer was 1.25 centimeters in diameter and superficial in depth. The RN took digital photographs of the ulcers and e-mailed them to an enterostomal therapist (wound care nurse specialist). The wound care nurse requested a team conference with the primary caregivers, and suggested that physical and occupational therapists join the treatment team. The physician approved these therapists.

68. Why do you think the RN took photographs of the ulcers?

____

____

____

You attend the team meeting and participate in care plan development. You are assigned to check the posterior tibial and dorsalis pedalis pulses daily and document your findings. You are to ask the patient about pain regularly and inform the RN if pain is present. The team agrees to meet weekly on Tuesdays to review the patient's progress.

69. Why is a daily posterior tibial and dorsalis pedalis pulse check important?

____

____

You will perform daily foam dressing changes to dry the wounds and control drainage. The goal is to reduce the pain, and the flat dressings will make it easier to apply antiembolism hosiery. You will measure the ulcers weekly or when there is a significant change in appearance and document your findings.

70. Why are wound measurements taken weekly?

71. What will you do if Mr. Rabb's wound measurements increase in size from one week to the next?

The occupational therapist taught Mrs. Rabb how to put on the antiembolism hosiery to reduce edema. You are to do the dressing change when she arrives each day, then work with her so that she becomes proficient in applying the hosiery. You notice a foul odor when you change the dressing, and inform the RN. She instructs you to obtain a wound culture.

72. What precautions will you take when doing the dressing changes?

The culture reveals an infection in the right leg, and Mr. Rabb is put on an antibiotic. The critical pathway calls for a progressive mobility program, with teaching and encouraging ADL independence with adaptive devices. You will walk Mr. Rabb to the activity room and back three times each day with a wheeled walker. The increased mobility was designed to stimulate circulation and improve the effectiveness of the compression stockings.

73. Why is ambulation important for this patient?

74. Mr. Rabb resists going to the activity room three times a day. He says he does not like the activities. What action will you take?

You recognize that Mrs. Rabb has great difficulty managing the antiembolism hosiery. Her husband is a large man, and she is petite and frail. She gets tears in her eyes and says she fears hurting her husband with pulling and tugging on the stockings. You mention this problem to the occupational therapist when she inquires about the patient. She considers an adaptive device, but subsequently does some additional research, and orders a new product that uses Velcro to secure the compression hosiery. The patient's wife manages these more easily, and within a week is proficient in applying them. She tells you that Mr. Rabb had a blood clot in his leg five years ago when they lived in another state. They subsequently moved to your town so a married daughter could assist them with Mr. Rabb's care. This is new information that you have not seen on any of the patient's records.

75. Is it important to notify anyone of this patient's past history of a blood clot? Why or why not? If yes, to whom will you report?

The ulcer begins to heal with the antibiotic, improved circulation, reduced edema, and foam dressings. The wound pain begins to subside. Mr. Rabb is discharged after four weeks of care, with the ulcer completely healed. A home health care agency will follow the patient at home to prevent ulcer recurrence. The agency worker is filling out a transfer form to give to the home care agency, and asks you for specific ADL information about the patient to put on the form. The RN stated that this was a tremendous accomplishment, and noted that the patient benefited from the team approach and frequent goal revisions.

76. What do you think caused the pain to subside?

77. Why did the team set goals for Mr. Rabb? Why are goals important?

78. How do the goals affect the patient's outcomes?

79. Why is it important to look at the patient as a whole rather than focusing strictly on the wound?

80. What type of information will you provide to the home health care agency?

81. Why is it important to share information with the home health care agency?

CHAPTER 6
Phlebotomy

ACTIVITIES

Vocabulary Exercise

Using the definitions provided, unscramble the words.

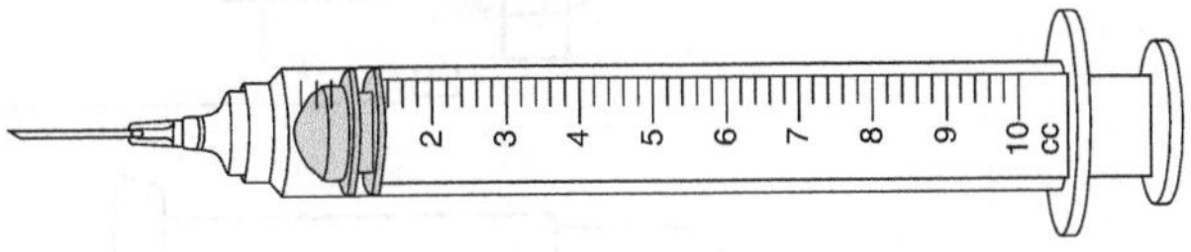

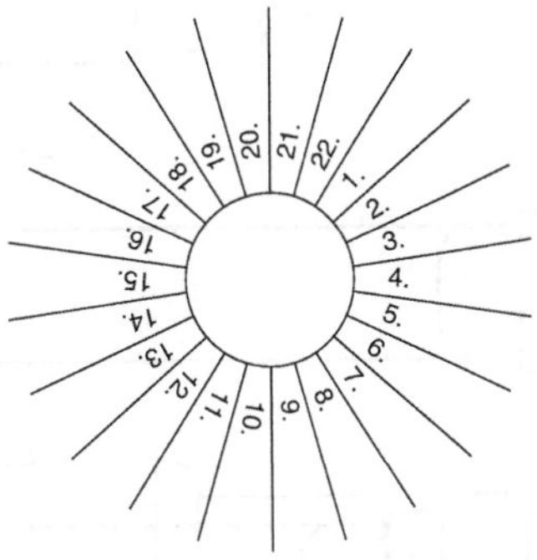

1. ymhobelopt
2. cunnievetupr
3. isbptohromhlebit
4. nemul
5. veleb
6. smolehsyi
7. uctainerva
8. yetbfutrl
9. noaguailtco
10. yeklyl
11. amehomat
12. cagnutioaantsl
13. latntecaubi space
14. oiquintetr
15. ceturlu
16. petsmiceia
17. robaeic
18. nobaaerci
19. microdraw
20. lacten
21. pillaracy tube
22. cifrugeten

1. **Collecting blood**
2. **Puncturing a vein with a needle**
3. **Inflammation of a vein with blood clot formation**
4. **Inside diameter of the needle**
5. **Slant or inclination at the end of a needle**
6. **Breaking of fragile blood cells**
7. **A vacuum tube**

(continues)

8. A winged infusion needle
9. Clotting of blood
10. A curved clamp with teeth
11. A blood-filled bruise, caused by the breaking of a blood vessel
12. Medications that prevent blood from clotting
13. Area in front of the elbow
14. A tight band that causes veins to fill with blood
15. A blood test to check for the presence of a systemic infection
16. A systemic blood infection
17. Pathogens that can live only in the presence of oxygen
18. Pathogens that live without oxygen
19. A small skin puncture used for collecting blood specimens
20. A tiny, sharp, sterile device used to puncture the skin to collect small blood samples
21. A slender, short, hollow tube that holds blood for laboratory testing
22. A device that holds and spins test tubes for laboratory testing

Labeling

Label the following diagrams.

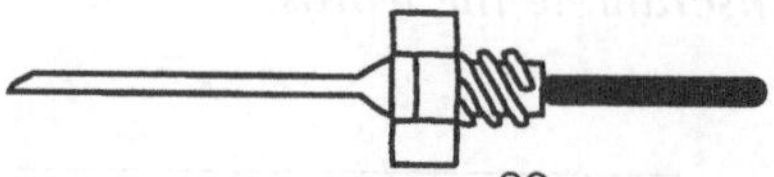

23. ____________________

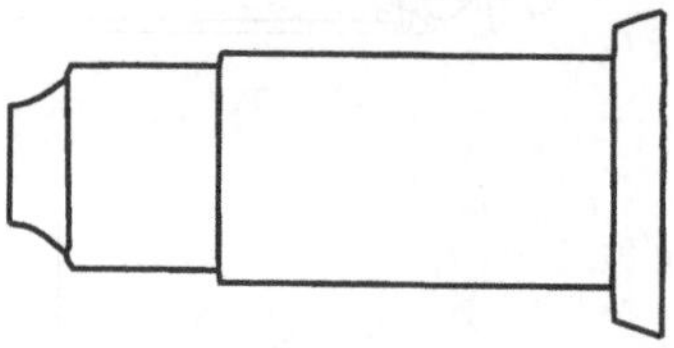

24. ____________________

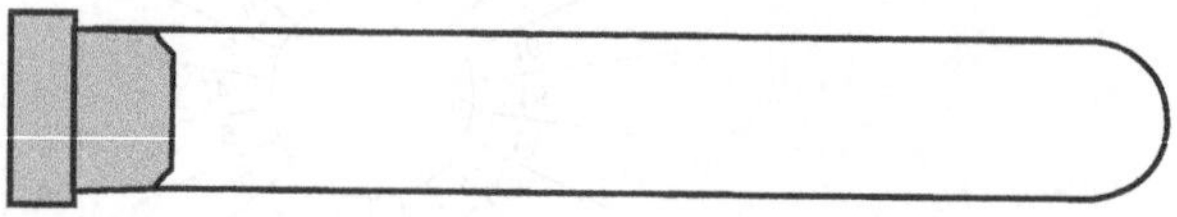

25. ____________________

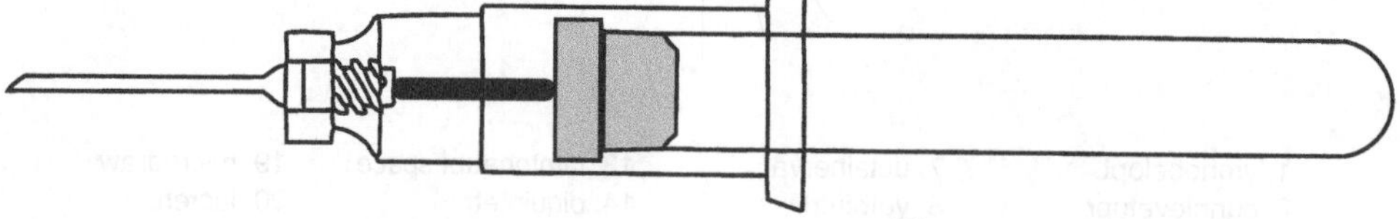

26. ____________________

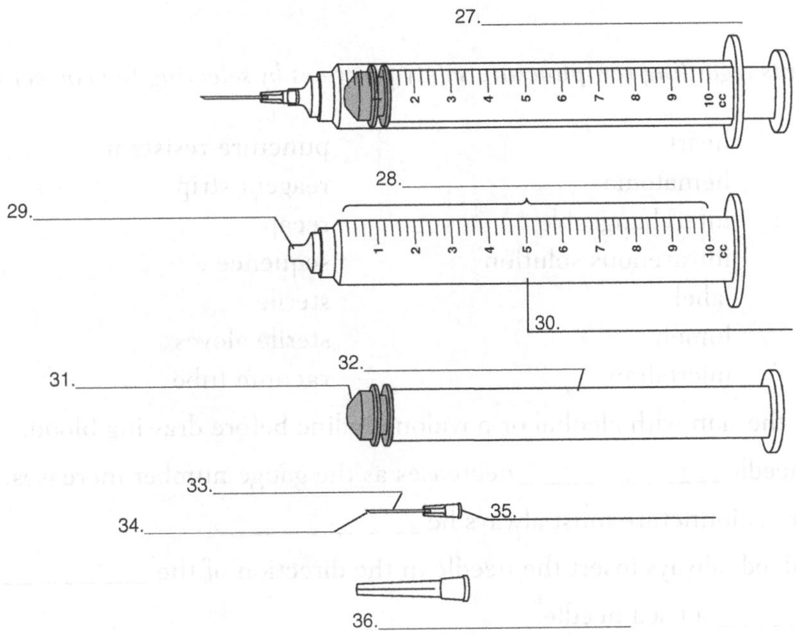

23. ______________________________
24. ______________________________
25. ______________________________
26. ______________________________
27. ______________________________
28. ______________________________
29. ______________________________
30. ______________________________
31. ______________________________
32. ______________________________
33. ______________________________
34. ______________________________
35. ______________________________
36. ______________________________

Completion

Complete the statements regarding venipuncture safety practices by selecting the correct term from the following list.

air	heart	puncture-resistant
arterial	hematoma	reagent strip
cleanse	interchangeable	recap
closed	intravenous solution	sequence
coagulate	label	sterile
elastic	lumen	sterile gloves
gauze pad	microdraw	vacuum tube

37. ______________ the skin with alcohol or povidone-iodine before drawing blood.
38. The size of the needle ______________ decreases as the gauge number increases.
39. Needles used for venipuncture must always be ______________.
40. When drawing blood, always insert the needle in the direction of the ______________.
41. Never ______________ a used needle.
42. Draw each test using the proper color tube, in the proper ______________.
43. Hold firm pressure over the insertion site with a ______________ ______________ while removing the needle.
44. Blood in the syringe will ______________ within 1 to 2 minutes after the specimen is collected.
45. Avoid drawing blood from an arm in which an ______________ ______________ is being administered.
46. The venous system is a ______________ system, filled with blood.
47. Accidentally injecting ______________ into the venous system has the potential to create serious problems.
48. Discard needles in a ______________-______________ container.
49. The most common complication of venipuncture is ______________.
50. Arteries are usually larger and more ______________ than veins.
51. Do not apply the tourniquet so tightly that it stops the ______________ blood flow.
52. The ______________-______________ method is the easiest and safest method to use for drawing blood.
53. The components of some vacuum systems are not ______________.
54. After performing a venipuncture, ______________ the tubes in the patient's room after collecting the specimen.
55. Because the blood culture is used to test for the presence of microbes, you should apply ______________ ______________ to prevent accidental contamination.
56. Blood drawn through a ______________ is a mixture of venous, capillary, and arterial blood.
57. When blood is collected from a lancet skin puncture, it is tested on a ______________ ______________ or is drawn into a capillary tube.

True/False

Circle T if the statement is true or F if it is false.

58. T F Use povidone-iodine to prep the skin when drawing a blood culture or test for blood alcohol.
59. T F Do not use a sterile package that is torn, damaged, has become wet, or is past the expiration date.

60. T F You may reuse an evacuated tube holder if a safety needle was used to draw blood.

61. T F Vacuum tubes will fill completely with blood.

62. T F Improper needle placement causes inability to draw blood despite having the needle in the vein.

63. T F Latex and iodine exposure during venipuncture is minimal, so allergies are not a consideration when drawing blood.

64. T F After you have finished drawing blood, instruct the patient to bend the arm up at the elbow.

65. T F Petechiae are tiny hemorrhagic spots, of pinpoint to pinhead size.

66. T F The median and basilic veins are the safest choice for drawing blood.

67. T F Tourniquets are a negligible source of transmission of infection.

68. T F Tourniquets that remain on limbs for extended periods of time can cause serious nerve and circulatory damage, leading to amputation.

69. T F Apply a bandage to the puncture site to stop bleeding.

70. T F Do not leave a tourniquet in place for more than five minutes.

71. T F If the patient feels dizzy or faint during the venipuncture procedure, stop.

72. T F When using the evacuated-tube system, blood cultures must be collected last.

73. T F Shake each test tube containing anticoagulant well to mix the blood specimen.

74. T F When drawing blood, needle length is determined by your personal preference.

75. T F Needles with a large diameter enable you to draw large volumes of blood quickly.

76. T F A vacutainer that is half full will usually provide enough blood to test the specimen.

77. T F If a needle is used to draw blood from small or collapsing veins, a butterfly needle is the safest method to use.

78. T F A coagulation tube has a red stopper.

Completion

Complete the table in the spaces provided.

Needle Type/Size	Suggested Use
79. 19 gauge	• ______________________
80. _____ gauge	• Consider using a butterfly, which is most comfortable for the patient • Commonly used for moderate to large veins, particularly those in the antecubital area • May be butterfly type or straight, multisample needle • May be used with butterfly or straight needle with vacutainer system or butterfly with syringe
81. 22 gauge	• ______________________ • Usually used to draw blood from antecubital area • Used to draw one to three tubes of blood
82. 23 gauge	• Most versatile and ______________ needle • Used for large to moderately small veins • May be used with straight, multisample needle with vacutainer system • May be used with butterfly with vacutainer system or butterfly with syringe

Needle Type/Size	Suggested Use
83. _____ gauge	• Used for smallest veins • Used for veins that collapse readily • Best used with a butterfly and syringe when drawing from small veins • Butterfly and vacutainer may be used if many tubes of blood are needed, but this increases the risk of vein collapse

Developing Greater Insight

Answer the following questions based on the situation described.

84. Before drawing blood, you will prepare the skin by wiping in the area of the proposed needle insertion site. Explain how to cleanse the area.

____

85. How large should the cleansed area be?

____

86. Should you wait for the skin to dry? Why or why not?

____

87. If povidone-iodine is used to cleanse the skin, how and when do you remove it?

____

88. Why is it removed in this manner?

____

89. Why do you hold pressure on the insertion site? Can the patient be instructed to do this? Why or why not?

____

90. Why is gauze used instead of cotton?

____

91. You must transfer blood from a syringe to an evacuated tube. Place the steps to the procedure in the correct order by labeling them with letters A through H.

_____ Label or sticker the tube of blood.

_____ The tube will fill until the vacuum is used. Do not depress the plunger to the syringe. This will cause hemolysis of the blood sample and increases the risk of blood spattering.

_____ Peel back the sterile package for the transfer device.

_____ With the syringe held vertically and the tip pointing down, center the tip of the vacutainer and press it up into the holder portion of the transfer device.

_____ Insert the tip of the syringe into the blood transfer device. Turn clockwise to secure.

_____ Engage the safety shield on the butterfly needle.

_____ Carefully remove the needle and place it in the sharps container.

_____ Separate the vacutainer tube from the transfer device and syringe. Discard the transfer device and syringe into the sharps container.

CHAPTER 7

Intravenous Therapy

ACTIVITIES

Vocabulary Exercise

1.–27. Fill in the words in the puzzle using the clues and definitions provided.

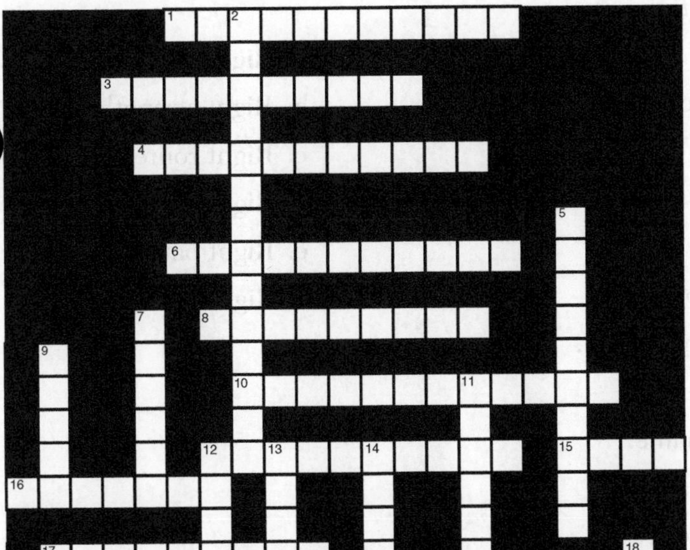

ACROSS

1. A _____ film dressing is commonly used to cover the insertion site.
3. _____ intravenous pumps regulate the flow of IV fluids electronically.
4. Intravenous administration of blood.
6. _____ therapy involves inserting a needle into a vein for the purpose of administering fluids and medications.
8. The _____ administration set is most commonly used for adults.
10. _____ occurs when the catheter or needle pierces the vein.
12. _____ are part of the immune system and serve as a protective mechanism against foreign materials.
15. The _____ mechanism provides a means of locking the tubing and needle or catheter together, making them more difficult to separate.
16. The _____ lock is a cap that covers the end, or hub, of the needle or catheter.
17. _____ is irritation of a vein caused by an IV device or medication.
19. A _____ intravenous catheter is a long catheter that is inserted into a vein in the shoulder or neck area and threaded through the venous system to the superior vena cava, or right atrium of the heart.

(continues)

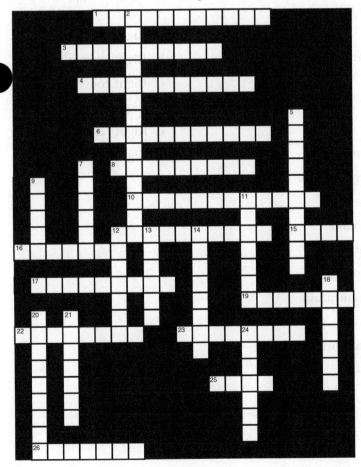

22. The _____ pin pierces the plastic IV bag or bottle.
23. An over-the-needle _____ is commonly used for short- or long-term IV therapy, and for restless patients.
25. The _____ control clamp is a roller clamp used to regulate the speed, or rate of fluid flow.
26. Intravenous containers are made of _____ materials.

DOWN

2. The _____ set has flexible, plastic tubing through which the solution flows; it is attached to the IV solution on one end and the patient on the other.
5. An IV _____ regulates gravity flow of IV fluids by counting drops of solution.
7. An inline _____ allows fluid to pass, but traps particles.
9. The lower _____ clamp is a plastic clamp used to stop or regulate the flow of fluid.
11. Strict _____ technique is used for starting and caring for an IV.
12. An _____ is a foreign substance that causes an allergic reaction.
13. The _____ test identifies the patient's blood type and Rh factor.
14. Fluid _____ occurs when fluids infuse too rapidly.
18. A child may be restrained by placing the child in a _____ board, and folding Velcro straps over the child's body.
20. The _____ administration set is most commonly used for children.
21. The drop _____ is the entry to the drop chamber.
24. Shearing the catheter tip off may create a catheter _____.

Matching

Label each of the following with the "right" for intravenous initiation and administration that applies to the statement. Each "right" may be used more than one time.

28. _____ Check the IV three times.
29. _____ Make sure the solution is labeled for IV use.
30. _____ Check the order for correct time.
31. _____ Never chart in advance.
32. _____ Always check the expiration date.
33. _____ Ask an RN to check your calculations.
34. _____ Make sure you have the correct preparation.
35. _____ Document dressing and tubing changes.
36. _____ Ask the patient to state his or her name.
37. _____ Place an I&O worksheet at the bedside.
38. _____ Compare the label to the MAR or order.
39. _____ Make sure you have the right concentration.
40. _____ Check for allergies.
41. _____ Document vital signs and other monitoring.
42. _____ Always check the patient's ID band.
43. _____ Initial the flow sheet promptly.
44. _____ Make sure all equipment is sterile.
45. _____ Use flawless sterile technique.

a. Right solution
b. Right strength
c. Right route
d. Right time
e. Right patient
f. Right documentation

True/False

Circle T if the statement is true or F if it is false.

46. T F Always select the macrodrip IV tubing unless directed otherwise by the RN.
47. T F A few small bubbles in the IV solution will not harm the patient.
48. T F Start the IV as low on the vein as possible.
49. T F Most IV infections are caused by pathogens that are already inside the patient's body.
50. T F The devices used for immobilizing IVs are not considered to be restraints.
51. T F Remove tape or transparent dressing by pulling in the direction of hair growth.
52. T F When using a controller, make sure the drip chamber is at least 30 inches above the insertion site.
53. T F Using an IV controller is as accurate as using a pump.
54. T F Pain and/or burning at the insertion site are symptoms of infiltration.
55. T F Peripheral intravenous catheters have the greatest risk of infection of all IVs.
56. T F Selection of the IV needle or catheter is determined by the length of IV therapy, type of solution, and condition of the veins.
57. T F Tape the junctions of the intravenous infusion system securely to prevent complications.
58. T F Use a permanent marker to write the time and your initials on the IV bottle.
59. T F Start the IV in the patient's dominant extremity, because the veins there are larger.
60. T F Start the IV with the bevel facing up.
61. T F Cover the needle or catheter insertion site well with tape.
62. T F Butterfly needles are useful for long-term IV therapy in children.
63. T F The rate of infection with metal needles is lower than with plastic catheters.
64. T F If you cannot find a suitable vein in the arms, check the patient's feet.
65. T F An infection is usually the result of phlebitis, rather than the cause.
66. T F Air embolus is a routine complication, and is usually not serious.

Labeling

Label the following diagram.

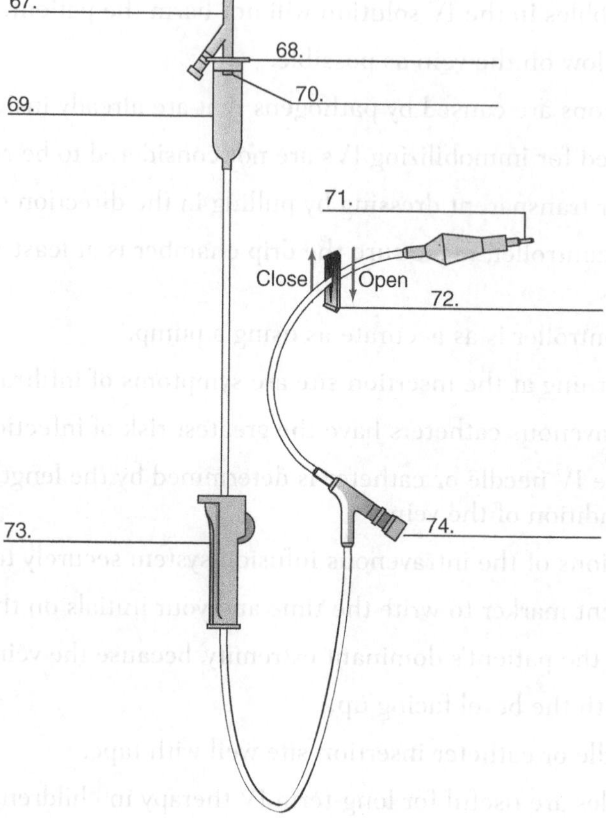

67. ______________________

68. ______________________

69. ______________________

70. ______________________

71. ______________________

72. ______________________

73. ______________________

74. ______________________

Developing Greater Insight

Review this case study from a medical malpractice lawsuit and answer the questions by identifying problems or potential problems, and then stating the correct actions to take.

A 34-year-old disabled female was admitted for treatment of influenza and vomiting. The patient alleged that the hospital personnel did not meet the standard of care because they started an IV in her foot, then administered an irritating anti-nausea medication into the IV. The patient stated that when the IV infiltrated, nursing personnel ignored her complaints of burning and pain, and continued the IV and medication administration. The patient stated that she had blanching discoloration from the ankle to the toes in the affected foot. She said that the IV was continued for another hour and 15 minutes after she registered her complaint, causing necrosis of the tissue and bone.

75. What is the standard of care for IV location? ____________________

76. What should have been done when the patient complained of burning and pain?

____

77. What do the signs and symptoms of burning, pain, and blanching of the foot suggest?

____

There was reportedly no documentation on the record of medication administration. An IV documentation was allegedly inadequate and incomplete. The patient contended that physician orders were written after nurses had already provided treatment. The hospital contended that these things were oversights, and that proper procedures had been followed. The hospital stated that the nurses had identified the IV infiltration in a timely manner and stopped the IV. The plaintiff contended that the IV should have been stopped immediately when she complained of burning and pain. She further alleged that nursing staff fell below the standard of care when they failed to follow the hospital's own policies, procedures, and guidelines in establishing an IV, and that they failed to adhere to proper policies regarding charting of treatment and administration of medications.

78. Is a physician order necessary to start an IV? ____________________

79. When should nursing personnel document that an IV was started?

____

80. What additional information should be documented regarding initiation of an IV?

____

____

81. If a PCT reports signs and symptoms such as burning, pain, and blanching to the RN, but the nurse fails to respond, what action should the PCT take?

____

____

____

The hospital denied liability, arguing that the plaintiff's condition was the result of the doctor's decision to start the IV and administer the medication. It contended that the doctor failed to intervene and treat the patient in a timely manner. It also claimed that the patient was at fault because she had informed personnel that she had previously had an IV started in her foot. The patient required nine surgeries to correct the damage, spent additional time in the hospital, and over a two-year period underwent multiple surgeries for irrigation, debridement, tendon removal, and ankle fusion. At the time of trial, she was facing the possibility of a below-the-knee amputation. A jury found in favor of the patient and awarded approximately $2.8 million in damages.

82. Who is responsible for monitoring an IV? ____________________

83. Who is responsible for informing the doctor of patient problems and that treatment is potentially needed?

____

84. This patient told nursing personnel that she had previously had an IV in her foot. What action would you take if a patient made a similar comment to you?

____

85. Where would you find information regarding hospital IV policies, procedures, and documentation?

CHAPTER 8

Urinary and Bowel Elimination

ACTIVITIES

Vocabulary Exercise

1.–38. *Fill in the words in the puzzle using the clues and definitions provided.*

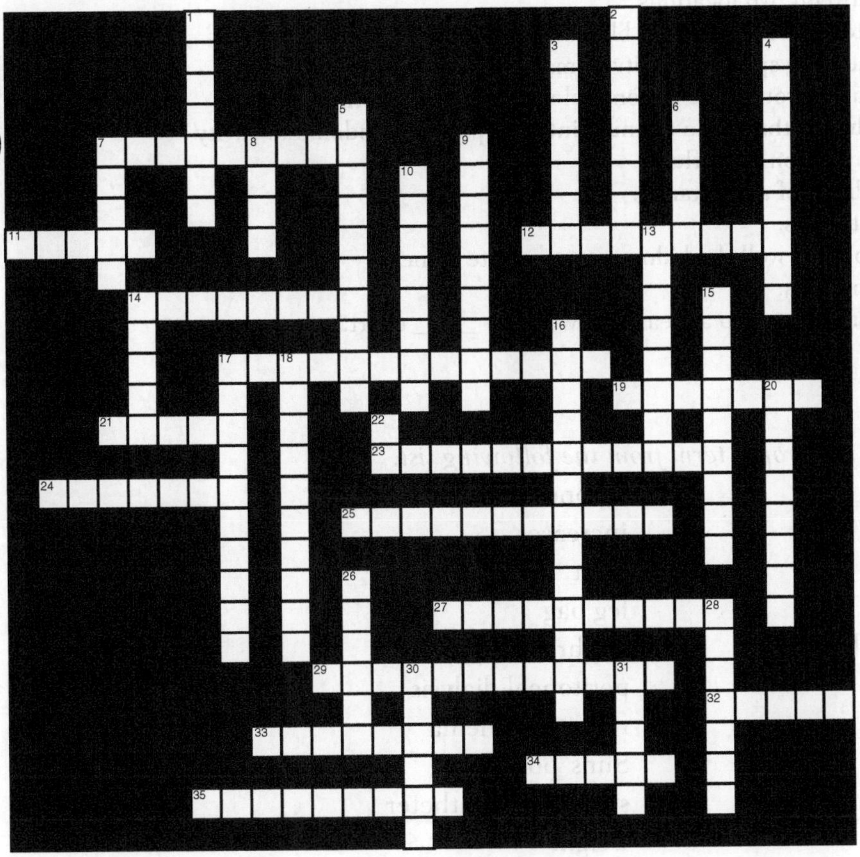

ACROSS

7. Patients with an indwelling catheter may complain of feeling the urge to urinate because of pressure of the balloon on the internal _____.
11. The introduction of fluid into the lower bowel to cleanse the anus, rectum, and lower colon.
12. Catheterization increases the risk of _____.
14. A _____ catheter is used to drain the bladder, and is immediately removed.
17. Rectal _____ may be given to stimulate bowel elimination.
19. A urinary catheter is inserted through the _____.
21. Always secure an indwelling catheter with a Velcro _____ or tape.
23. _____ involves the use of a machine to clean wastes from the blood after the kidneys have failed.

24. The most desirable form of dialysis access, created by connecting an artery to a vein in the arm.
25. A _____ tube is surgically inserted through the skin and into the kidney to drain urine directly to the outside of the body.
27. An _____ catheter remains in the bladder.
29. A urinary catheter should never be used as a treatment for _____.
32. Stimulating the _____ nerve will slow the heart rate.
33. A tube that is inserted into the bladder to drain urine.
34. Always keep the urinary drainage bag _____ the level of the bladder.
35. The most common type of ostomy; located between the colon and the abdomen.

DOWN

1. Always use _____ technique when inserting or caring for a catheter.
2. A gland that is often problematic in elderly males. It surrounds the urethra just below the bladder, and secretes fluid in semen.
3. A catheter is held in place in the bladder by an inflatable _____.
4. The ostomy _____ is the plastic container into which the contents of the bowel are emptied.
5. Bladder _____ is a treatment used when obstructions such as blood clots are present.
6. A piece of plastic tubing that is surgically inserted and connects an artery to a vein.
7. A surgically created opening into the body.
8. Continuous Ambulatory Peritoneal Dialysis.
9. Fecal _____ is the most serious form of constipation.
10. A procedure to cleanse the blood of toxins and impurities when the kidneys have failed.
13. In some _____, the female's body must be covered when members of opposite gender are present.
14. A connector to allow blood flow between two locations.
15. The _____ test checks urine for ketones, bilirubin, and blood, among other things.
16. A handheld unit that is used for checking specific gravity in many facilities.
17. A _____ catheter is inserted surgically through the abdominal wall directly into the bladder.
18. _____ dialysis involves inserting solution through a cannula into the patient's abdominal cavity.
20. Chemicals used to perform certain tests on body fluids.
22. An indication of the acidity or alkalinity of a substance.
26. The type of scale used for sizing catheters.
28. Urine specific _____ is a measure of how well the kidneys concentrate urine.
30. A surgically created opening into the body.
31. Check your findings by comparing the test strip appearance with the _____ chart.

Completion

Complete each statement by filling in the proper term from the following list.

bowel movement
chemical burns
cleansing enema
commercially prepared enemas
continuous ambulatory peritoneal dialysis
encourage fluids
fecal impaction
female
flatus
function
horizontally
incontinence
increases
least
leg bag
nephrostomy tube
peritoneal dialysis
retention enema
Sims' position
suprapubic catheter
weight

39. The pH of the urine provides information about the _______________ of the kidneys.
40. When testing urine with a multiple-test reagent strip, hold the strip _______________ while it is processing.

41. As urine becomes more concentrated, the specific gravity ____________.
42. The risk of urinary infection from a catheter is highest in ____________ patients.
43. Inform the RN if the patient does not have a ____________ ____________ in three days.
44. A patient with ____________ ____________ may have loose stools, giving the impression of diarrhea.
45. Change the ostomy appliance 2 to 4 hours after meals, because this is the time when the bowel is ____________ active.
46. Some reagents will cause ____________ ____________ if handled with wet hands.
47. With patients who have cognitive impairments, ____________ is often a communication problem, not a physical problem.
48. When caring for a catheterized patient, you should ____________ ____________.
49. Avoid putting the patient to bed when wearing a ____________ ____________.
50. Headache and profuse sweating are signs and symptoms of a plugged ____________ ____________.
51. The ____________ ____________ drains urine continuously.
52. Patients receiving dialysis usually have orders for daily ____________.
53. ____________ ____________ involves inserting dialysis solution through a cannula into the patient's abdominal cavity.
54. ____________ ____________ is a type of dialysis that the patient may do at home.
55. The rectal tube is used to eliminate ____________.
56. A ____________ ____________ removes fecal material from the rectum and lower bowel, stimulates peristalsis, and softens stool.
57. A ____________ ____________ is usually an oil-based solution.
58. ____________ ____________ are administered in small, premeasured containers.
59. The ____________ ____________ is a side-lying position used for giving enemas, doing rectal examinations, and performing other rectal treatments.

Short Answer

Write the information in the space provided.

60. List 10 guidelines for reagent strip testing.
    a. ____________
    b. ____________
    c. ____________
    d. ____________
    e. ____________
    f. ____________
    g. ____________
    h. ____________
    i. ____________
    j. ____________

61. List 10 guidelines for caring for a patient who uses a catheter.

a. ______

b. ______

c. ______

d. ______

e. ______

f. ______

g. ______

h. ______

i. ______

j. ______

62. List five guidelines for opening a closed drainage system.

a. ______

b. ______

c. ______

d. ______

e. ______

63. List 10 guidelines for applying a urinary leg bag.

a. ______

b. ______

c. ______

d. ______

e. ______

f. ______

g. ______

h. ______

i. ______

j. ______

Procedure Review

Using a crayon or colored pencil, label the following peritoneal dialysis diagram. Write the names of each part on the corresponding line.

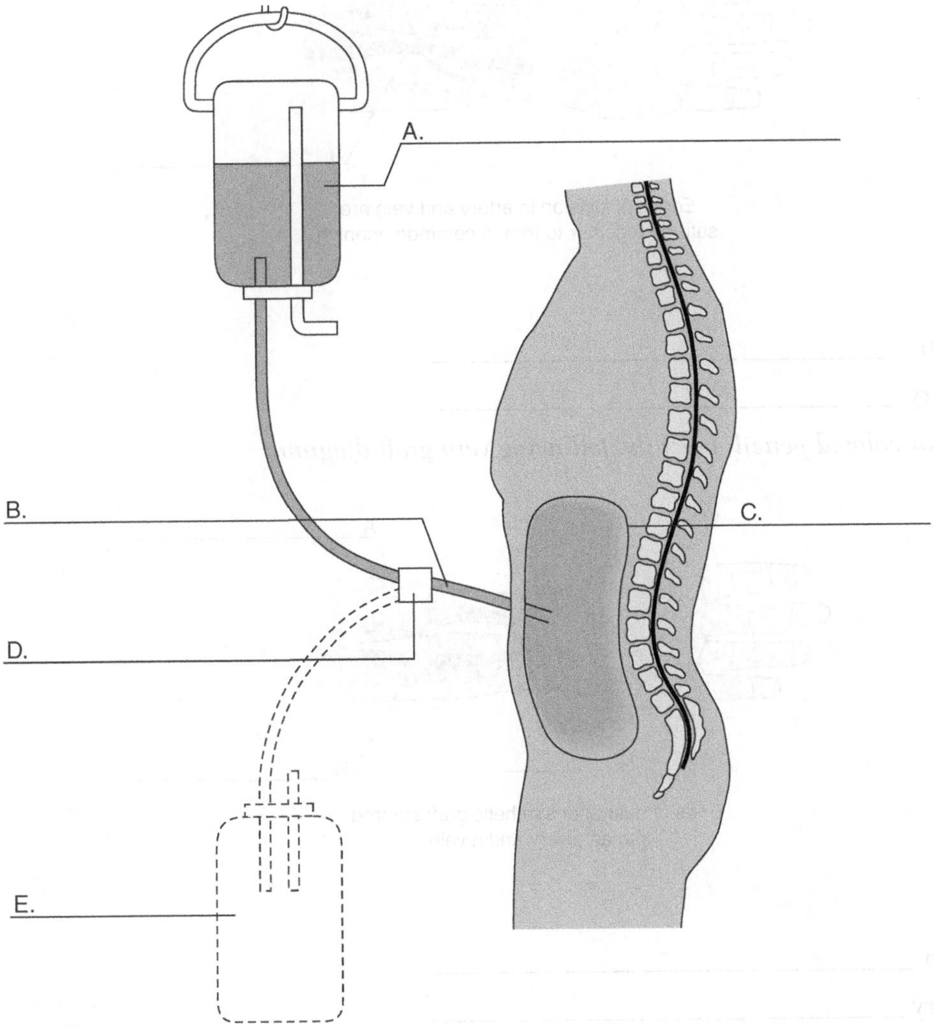

Blue—peritoneal cavity
Red—draw arrows for the flow of fresh dialysate into the peritoneum
Green—draw arrows for the flow of dialysate solution that has filtered impurities
Purple—peritoneal clamp
Pink—peritoneal catheter
Orange—waste container

64.

A. ______________________________

B. ______________________________

C. ______________________________

D. ______________________________

E. ______________________________

Using a crayon or colored pencil, label the following AV fistula diagram.

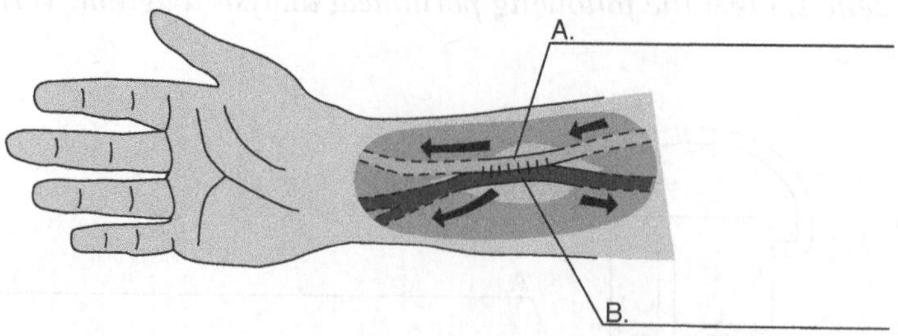

Edges of incision in artery and vein are sutured together to form a common opening.

65.

A. Blue—vein ________________

B. Red—artery ________________

Using a crayon or colored pencil, label the following vein graft diagram.

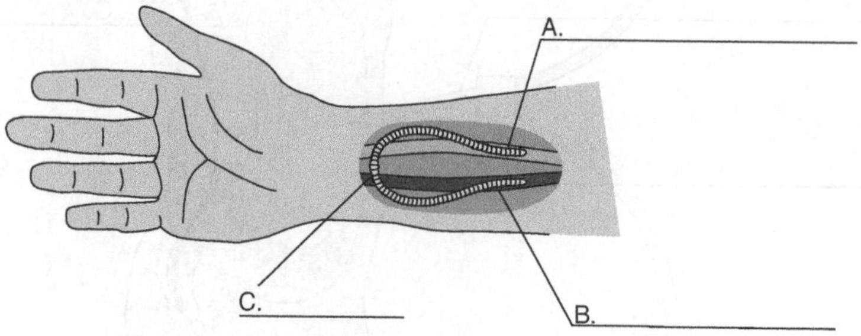

Ends of natural or synthetic graft sutured into an artery and a vein.

66.

A. Blue—vein ________________

B. Red—artery ________________

C. Green—synthetic graft material sutured in place ________________

Identify the parts of the colostomy bag.

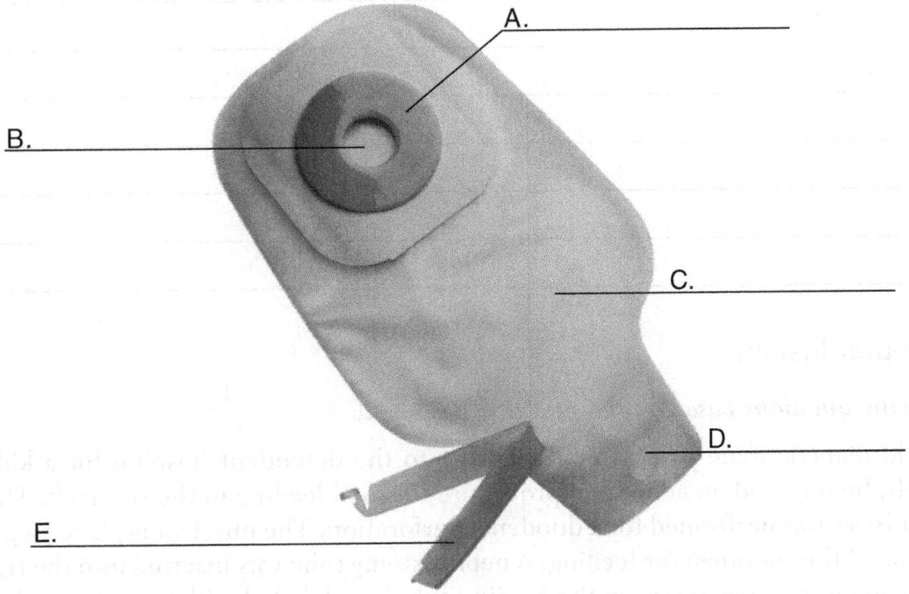

67.

A. ______________________

B. ______________________

C. ______________________

D. ______________________

E. ______________________

Identification

Carefully study the picture and identify 7 barriers to aiding the resident's normal elimination pattern.

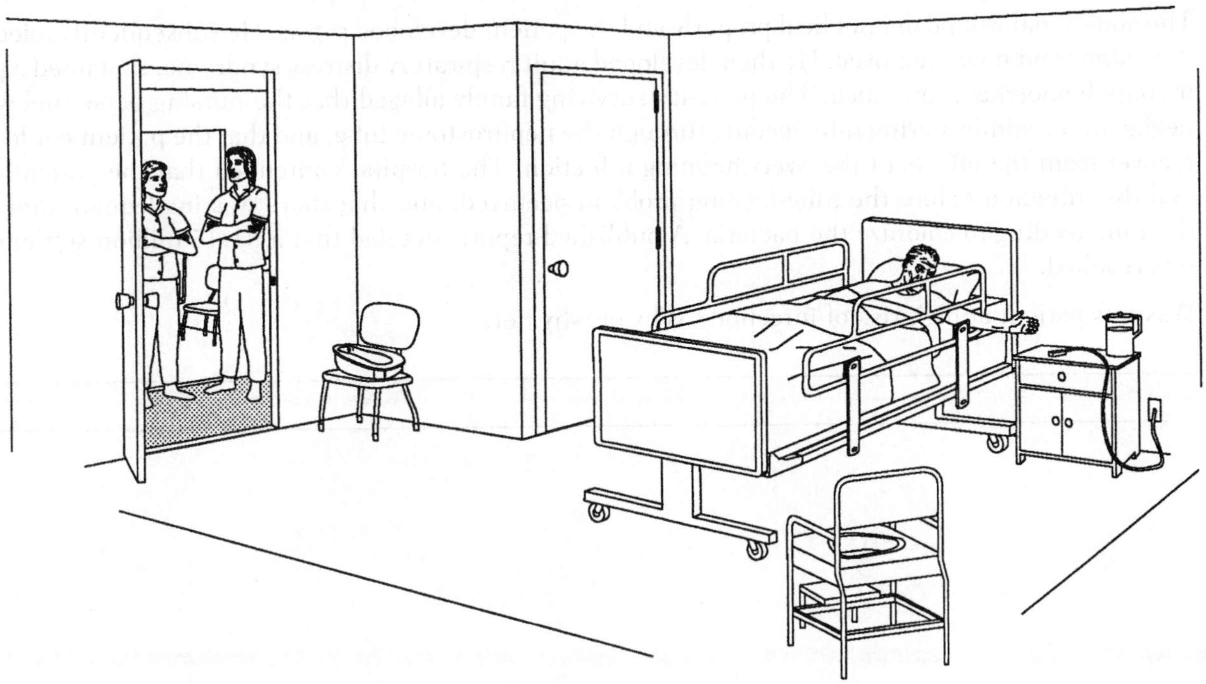

68.

Developing Greater Insight

Answer the following questions based on the situation described.

A 62-year-old diabetic male patient was admitted to the defendant hospital for a kidney transplant. Subsequently, he required an additional procedure to stop bleeding in the stomach. The following day, additional surgery was performed for a duodenal perforation. The physicians placed a gastrostomy tube in the left side of the abdomen for feeding. A nephrostomy tube was inserted into the right kidney. Both tubes were similar in appearance, so the feeding tube was labeled with tape. Several days later, nursing personnel inadvertently administered the tube feeding into the nephrostomy tube. A physician identified the problem within four hours, and immediately took the patient to the operating room to cleanse and remove the feeding material. Culture and sensitivity testing from this procedure revealed the presence of *Streptococcus, Enterobacter,* and *Acinetobacter,* hospital-acquired pathogens.

69. When a patient has multiple tubes, how do you identify the purpose of each?

70. What action can the PCT take to ensure that a tube feeding is not inadvertently administered into the wrong tube?

The abdominal wound did not heal properly and the patient developed sepsis. He subsequently rejected the kidney and it was removed. He then developed adult respiratory distress syndrome, sustained a pulmonary hemorrhage, and died. The patient's surviving family alleged that the nursing personnel were negligent for administering tube feeding through the nephrostomy tube, and that the patient could not recover from the effects of the overwhelming infection. The hospital contended that the patient had had the infection before the tube-feeding problem occurred, and that there was inadequate time for the tube feeding to colonize the bacteria. A published report revealed that a $1.45 million settlement was reached.

71. Was this patient at high risk of infection? Why or why not?

72. What general infection control measures would you use when caring for an elderly transplant patient who had had multiple surgeries, and had a feeding tube, nephrostomy tube, IV, and open surgical wounds?

____

____

73. Where would you look for guidance in how to care for this patient?

____

____

CHAPTER 9
Enteral Nutrition

ACTIVITIES

Vocabulary Exercise

1.–16. Fill in the words in the puzzle using the clues and definitions provided.

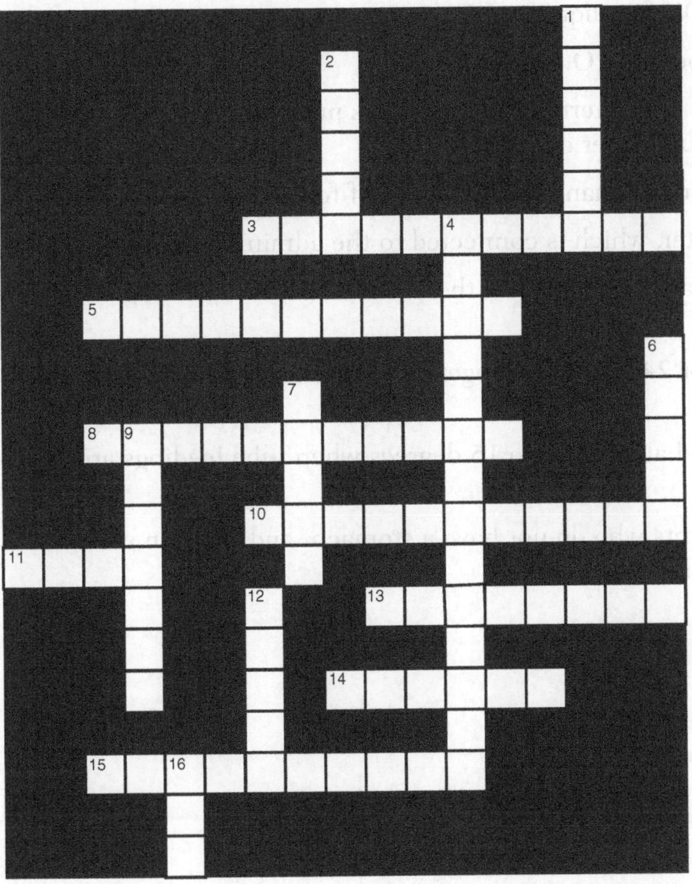

ACROSS

3. A _____ tube is inserted through the nose and threaded through the esophagus to the stomach.
5. A _____ tube is surgically inserted through the abdominal wall into the stomach.
8. A very serious inflammation of the peritoneum, the membrane that lines the abdominal cavity.
10. A _____ drape has a hole in the center.
11. Never place _____ food coloring into the tube-feeding solution.
13. *Clostridium difficile* causes _____.
14. A modified _____ swallow is done to identify the need for a feeding tube.
15. Inhalation of food and fluids into the lungs

DOWN

1. Buried _____ syndrome is an ulceration of the tissue at the feeding-tube exit site or the internal mucosal layer of the gastric wall.
2. _____ feeding is an intermittent method of feeding with a syringe.
4. Drip and pump feedings are given through an _____ set.
6. Tube-feeding formulas are approximately 15% _____ material.
7. Never use a _____ catheter in place of a feeding tube.
9. Feeding tubes are commonly called _____ tubes.

(continues)

12. Patients receiving tube feedings also require additional _____ each day.
16. A _____ tube is surgically inserted by the physician by using an endoscope. The tube is threaded down the esophagus and exits through an incision in the abdomen over the stomach.

True/False

Circle T if the statement is true or F if it is false.

17. T F A nasogastric tube is usually used when the patient will require tube feeding for a short period of time.
18. T F The registered dietitian closely follows all patients who use feeding tubes.
19. T F Blue food coloring is routinely added to tube feedings to help personnel identify vomitus and oral secretions.
20. T F A gastrostomy feeding button is a short-term device.
21. T F Gastrostomy tubes are routinely changed every 30 days.
22. T F The external PEG bumper should fit tightly against the skin.
23. T F A misplaced feeding tube or Foley catheter used in place of a gastrostomy tube may migrate and cause peritonitis.
24. T F Patients who are getting tube feedings cannot become dehydrated.
25. T F Enteral formulas are considered 100% free liquid.
26. T F Patients with feeding tubes should be on I&O.
27. T F Undue tension between the internal and external PEG bumpers promotes ulceration and migration of the tube into the muscular layer of the stomach.
28. T F Feeding bags must be filled with no more than 8 hours' worth of formula.
29. T F A PEG tube is plugged into an adapter, which is connected to the administration set.
30. T F When you hang a tube feeding, use a marker to write the date and time on the bag or other container of formula.
31. T F A closed-system feeding can hang for 24 hours, or longer as recommended by the manufacturer.
32. T F The head of the bed must be elevated at least 10 to 15 degrees when tube feedings are administered.
33. T F Jejunostomy tubes are used for patients who do not have a stomach, and those in whom recurrent formula aspiration is a problem.

Completion

Complete the following table.

Body Fluid	pH
34. stomach contents	_____ to _____
35. intestinal contents	_____ to _____
36. respiratory secretions	usually _____ or higher

Short Answer

Write the information in the space provided.

37. Explain why it is necessary to check tube-feeding placement.

38. State when you should check tube-feeding placement.

39. List four methods of checking tube-feeding placement.

a.

b.

c.

d.

40. Discuss why it is important to elevate the head of the bed when tube feedings are being administered.

Using a crayon or colored pencil, label the following diagram.

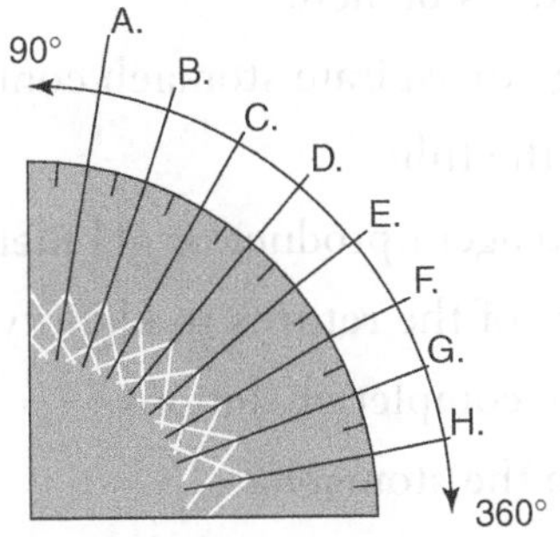

Blue—lowest level of elevation of bed when tube feeding is running

Red—highest recommended level of elevation of bed when tube feeding is running

Label the degrees in the diagram.

41.

A. ______________________________

B ______________________________

C. ______________________________

D. ______________________________

E. ______________________________

F. ______________________________

G. ______________________________

H. ______________________________

42. What effect does elevating the patient's head have on the patient's skin condition, and what PCT measures can be taken to reduce the risk?

____

____

____

43. State why the head of the bed should remain elevated for at least one hour after tube-feeding administration is completed.

____

____

____

You must check nasogastric tube placement before initiating a feeding. Place the steps to the procedure in the correct order by labeling them with numbers 1 through 10.

44.

_____ Return the aspirate to the stomach.

_____ Pull back on the syringe to aspirate stomach contents.

_____ Remove the plug from the tube.

_____ Check the pH using a reagent product or pH meter.

_____ Observe the appearance of the returns to identify gastric fluid.

_____ Perform your procedure completion actions.

_____ Inject 20 mL of air into the stomach.

_____ Perform your beginning procedure actions.

_____ Insert the syringe into the nasogastric tube.

_____ Replace the plug into the tube.

45. Explain how to check tube feeding for residual.

____

____

46. What should you do with the stomach contents after removing fluid to check residual?

____

____

47. Describe how to determine whether to proceed with tube feeding based on the amount of feeding residual.

____

____

48. You enter a patient's room and find her vomiting. The patient has a gastrostomy tube feeding running. When you added the formula to the continuous drip administration set, the patient's head was elevated. She apparently used the electric bed control to lower the head of the bed, and she is lying flat on her back. List the three most important PCT actions to take.

a. ____

b. ____

c. ____

Developing Greater Insight

Answer the following questions based on the situation described.

You enter Mr. Tinsley's room at the beginning of your shift when you are making rounds. The patient has a continuous gastrostomy tube feeding through a pump. When you check the pump settings, you discover that Jevity is infusing into the tube. You learned in report that the patient is a brittle, insulin-dependent diabetic who has an order for Glucerna in his gastrostomy tube. The patient appears to be sleeping. He is snoring loudly, and is difficult to arouse. When you succeed in awakening him, he is confused. His skin is hot and dry to touch, and his pulse is bounding.

49. What action will you take first?

____

50. What will you do next?

____

51. What monitoring will you do for this patient during your shift?

____

52. Is an incident report necessary?

____

CHAPTER 10
Specimen Collection

ACTIVITIES

Vocabulary Exercise

Find the words in the puzzle. If the word is part of a phrase, only the words in italics are hidden in the puzzle. Define each word or phrase.

a	O	l	n	o	s	o	c	o	m	i	a	l	t	g	c
e	m	g	a	x	d	j	k	n	a	l	f	c	l	a	k
x	t	e	c	n	M	s	C	S	y	a	i	u	l	g	y
p	r	s	h	o	c	p	f	r	M	l	c	c	S	l	t
e	a	y	Y	t	l	e	U	C	o	o	u	a	p	y	i
c	n	s	X	e	y	o	t	c	s	l	n	R	t	c	v
t	s	t	M	D	N	r	n	e	i	o	O	E	D	a	i
o	p	e	t	O	T	u	e	i	i	w	y	t	S	t	t
r	o	m	d	U	A	o	a	t	z	s	w	S	B	e	i
a	r	i	c	P	c	n	a	m	e	a	p	v	S	d	s
t	t	c	f	c	a	r	d	e	J	r	t	u	F	z	n
e	n	s	u	l	b	K	z	V	B	q	u	i	t	Q	e
t	x	l	y	i	s	w	a	b	g	P	P	t	o	u	s
J	t	s	l	p	r	a	n	d	i	a	l	Y	l	n	m
E	i	a	i	D	m	a	e	r	t	s	d	i	m	u	Z
s	c	r	e	q	u	i	s	i	t	i	o	n	x	s	c

1. gastric *analysis* ____
2. renal *calculi* ____
3. calibration ____
4. renal *colic* ____
5. colonization ____

(continues)

6. culture ______________________________
7. erythematic ______________________________
8. expectorate ______________________________
9. flank ______________________________
10. FSBS ______________________________
11. blood *glucose* ______________________________
12. *glycated* hemoglobin ______________________________
13. Lancet ______________________________
14. *midstream* urinalysis ______________________________
15. *nosocomial* infection ______________________________
16. *occult* blood ______________________________
17. 2-hour post*prandial* sugar ______________________________
18. laboratory *requisition* ______________________________
19. sensitivity ______________________________
20. sputum ______________________________
21. swab ______________________________
22. *systemic* infection ______________________________
23. *transport* bag ______________________________

Matching

Match the test name with the proper test type or test characteristics.

24. _____	identifies pathogens in fluids, wounds, etc.	a. catheterized urine specimen
25. _____	checks for acid in stomach	b. ova and parasites
26. _____	urine collected from middle of the stream	c. glucometer
27. _____	urine test for hormones, electrolytes, proteins	d. Group A *Streptococcus*
28. _____	sterile urine specimen to check for infection	e. midstream urine
29. _____	stool specimen tested for blood	f. wound culture and sensitivity
30. _____	fingerstick blood sugar	g. pediatric urine specimen
31. _____	checks blood sugar after a meal	h. culture and sensitivity
32. _____	throat swab	i. strain urine
33. _____	zigzag wound swab	j. postprandial blood sugar
34. _____	test for kidney stones	k. gastric analysis
35. _____	self-adhesive collection device	l. glycated hemoglobin
36. _____	stool specimen X3	m. 24-hour urine
37. _____	blood sugar over past 90 days	n. Hemoccult

True/False

Circle T if the statement is true or F if it is false.

38. T F Apply the principles of contact precautions when collecting laboratory specimens.
39. T F Swab cultures are always collected using a cotton culturette.
40. T F Specimens for culture testing are always collected in sterile containers.
41. T F When a patient has a catheter, the urine specimen is collected from the drainage bag.
42. T F Blood is present in the stool if the reagent in the Hemoccult test turns green.
43. T F The postprandial blood sugar is collected 4 hours after a meal.
44. T F A colonized wound will not heal until the infection is resolved.
45. T F Pressure ulcers seldom become colonized with bacteria.
46. T F Wounds are cultured routinely.
47. T F Erythema is increasing, abnormal redness and inflammation due to capillary congestion.
48. T F Renal calculi are tiny in size, but are very painful for the patient.
49. T F An infection is generally considered nosocomial if it occurs 48 hours or more after a hospital admission.
50. T F Bloodborne pathogens may be transmitted on an unclean glucose meter.
51. T F Glycated hemoglobin is a measurement of glucose over a four-month period of time.
52. T F A systemic infection spreads throughout the whole body.
53. T F Group A *Streptococcus pyogenes* causes rheumatic fever and kidney damage.
54. T F Culture testing is done to identify pathogens.
55. T F Sensitivity testing is done to identify antibiotics that eliminate the identified pathogen.
56. T F A sputum specimen analyzes saliva from the mouth.
57. T F The gastric analysis checks for the presence of pathogens in the stomach.
58. T F A nasogastric tube must be inserted to obtain a gastric analysis.
59. T F The normal blood sugar is between 65 and 120; in most facilities the value is 70 to 110.
60. T F Routine collection of a urine specimen from a child without bladder control is accomplished by using a straight catheter.
61. T F In persons without diabetes, the normal A1C value is approximately 7.0 percent.
62. T F In persons with diabetes, the normal A1C value is approximately 5.0 percent.
63. T F When collecting a swab specimen for Gram stain, do not break the ampule in the bottom of the culturette.
64. T F The patient should be NPO for 8 hours before the A1C test is collected.
65. T F Collect a throat culture by swabbing the base of the tongue and roof of the mouth.
66. T F Pathogens in the wound compete for the substances needed for healing.
67. T F If wound healing does not occur, the patient's entire treatment plan will be reviewed.
68. T F The first morning void is preferred for a midstream specimen.

Completion

You must analyze a stool specimen using the Hemoccult test. Place the steps to the procedure in the correct order by labeling them A through M.

69.

_____ Apply a thin layer of stool on panel one.

_____ Perform your procedure completion actions.

_____ Provide privacy until the patient has a bowel movement. Tell him or her to signal when finished, and return promptly.

_____ Within 60 seconds, compare the results with the color changes described on the package. If the sample turns blue, this suggests the presence of blood.

_____ Apply gloves.

_____ Perform your beginning procedure actions.

_____ Using the tongue blade, collect a small amount of stool.

_____ Apply 2 drops of developing solution on each panel of stool, and to the control at the bottom of the slide.

_____ Assist the patient with cleaning the perineum, handwashing, and returning to bed, as necessary.

_____ Turn the package over.

_____ Assist the patient with the bedpan or commode, or position the specimen collection device in the toilet.

_____ Obtain a second small specimen from a different part of the stool. Apply a thin layer to panel two.

_____ Lift the flap.

The three enemies of specimen collection are time, temperature, and desiccation. Explain PCT considerations to prevent these problems from occurring.

70. Time ____

71. Temperature ____

72. Desiccation ____

Developing Greater Insight

Answer the following questions based on the situation described.

Most lab tests are ordered by computer. However, when the computer is down, you must order the labs by hand. The doctors make rounds and order labs on their patients. Use the laboratory requisition forms in the figures to order tests on these patients.

73. Mrs. Estella A. Hernandez (routine labs)

Hospital number HE938668

Room 438B

Date: June 1

Physician: B. Smith

Collection times: June 2 AM routine

CMP (complete metabolic profile, comprehensive chemistry)

CBC (complete blood count)

Urinalysis

LABORATORY REQUISITION I

HOSPITAL NO ________ ROOM NO ____ DATE ______
NAME (LAST) ________ FIRST ________ MI ____
ADDRESS ________________________
PHYSICIAN ________________________

CHECK SECTIONS ORDERED

___ PROFILES	___ COAGULATION	___ HEMATOLOGY
___ CHEMISTRY	___ URINE TESTS	___ BLOOD BANK
___ SPEC. CHEM.	___ SEROLOGY	___ MISC.

ORDERING INFORMATION

DATE REQUESTED ___/___/___ TIME ORDERED ______ ___ AM ___ PM
DATE TO BE DRAWN (IF DIFFERENT THAN ABOVE) ________
___ ROUTINE ___ ASAP
___ STAT ___ TIMED ________ ___ AM ___ PM

COLLECTION INFORMATION

COLLECTED BY ________________________
DATE COLLECTED ___/___/___ TIME COLLECTED ______ AM ___ PM
SPECIMEN SOURCE ___ VEIN ___ CAP ___ OTHER (SPECIFY) ___
COMMENTS ________________________

PROFILES

___ ELECTROLYTES
___ CHEMISTRY 7, METABOLIC
___ CHEMISTRY COMPREHENSIVE
___ CARDIAC PROFILE
___ FOLLOW-UP (8–12 hrs.)
___ FOLLOW-UP (2nd day)
___ LIVER PROFILE
___ THYROID PROFILE
___ LIPID PROFILE
___ GLUCOSE TOLERANCE TEST HRS ___

CHEMISTRY

TEST	RESULTS	RES. VALUES	
___ SODIUM	______	(135-153)	MEQ/L
___ POTASSIUM	______	(3.5-5.3)	MEQ/L
___ CHLORIDE	______	(98-109)	MEQ/L
___ TOTAL CO2	______	(24-31)	MEQ/L
___ GLUCOSE	______	(70-110)	MG/DL
___ BUN	______	(8-23)	MG/DL
___ CREATININE	______	(0.5-1.5)	MG/DL
___ GGTP	______	(7-64)	U/L
___ SGPT (ALT)	______	(10-60)	U/L
___ SGOT (AST)	______	(10-42)	U/L
___ ALK PHOS	______	(26-88)	U/L
___ LDH	______	(91-180)	U/L
___ CPK	______	(22-269)	U/L
___ TRIGLYCERIDES	______	(10-190)	MG/DL
___ CHOLESTEROL	______	(133-240)	MG/DL
___ T-BILIRUBIN	______	(<1.0)	MG/DL
___ URIC ACID	______	(2.5-7.7)	MG/DL
___ PHOSPHORUS	______	(2.5-4.8)	MG/DL
___ CALCIUM	______	(8.5-10.1)	MG/DL
___ TOTAL PROT.	______	(6.0-8.5)	G/DL
___ ALBUMIN	______	(3.5-5.5)	G/DL
___ AMYLASE	______	(44-128)	U/L
___ D-BILIRUBIN	______	(<0.3)	MG/DL
___ CKMB	______	(<5%)	U/L
___ MAGNESIUM	______	(1.6-3.0)	MG/DL
___ ______			
___ ______			
___ ______			

COAGULATION

TEST	RESULTS	REF. VALUES
___ PROTIME (PT)	______	PATIENT SEC.
	______	CONTROL SEC.
___ APTT (PTT)	______	PATIENT SEC.
	______	CONTROL SEC.
___ FIBRINOGEN	______	(200-400) MG/DL
___ FDP	______	(<10) MCG/DL
___ THROMBIN TIME	______	(11-13) SEC.
___ BLEEDING TIME	______	(2.3-9.5) MIN.

URINE TESTS

TEST	RESULTS	REF. VALUES
___ URINALYSIS	______	
___ PREGNANCY TEST	______	
___ CREATININE CLEARANCE	______	M 70-160 ML/MIN F 78-115 ML/MIN
URINE CREAT.	______	MG/DL M 1.0-2.0 G/24HR F 0.8-1.8 G/24HR
URINE PROT. 24 HOUR	______	(<165) MB/24HR

SPECIAL CHEMISTRY

TEST	RESULTS	REF. VALUES
___ T3 UPTAKE	______	(23-34) %
___ T4	______	(4.5-12.0) UG/DL
___ T7 (FTI)	______	(1.0-4.0)
___ DIGOXIN	______	(0.8-2.0) MG/DL
___ THEOPHYLLINE	______	(10-20) UG/ML
___ PHENYTON	______	(10-20) UG/ML
___ PHENOBARB	______	(15-40) UG/ML
___ GENTAMICIN	______	( ) PK/TR
___ TORBRAMYCIN	______	( ) PK/TR
___ ALCOHOL	______	Toxic > 100 MG/DL
___ CARBAMAZEPHINE	______	(8-12) UG/ML
___ QUINIDINE	______	(2-5) UG/ML
___ NAPA	______	(2-8) UG/ML
___ PROCAINAMIDE	______	(4-8) UG/ML
___ ACETAMINOPHEN	______	(<200) UG/ML
___ LIDOCAINE	______	(1.2-5) MG/ML
___ SALICYLATE	______	(100-200) MG/L
___ LITHIUM	______	(0.5-1.0)
___ DRUG SCREEN	______	SENT TO REF LAB
___ ______		
___ ______		
___ ______		

HEMATOLOGY

___ CBC
___ MANUAL DIFF.
___ HEMOGRAM (Hgb. & Hct.)
___ RETIC. COUNT
___ SED. RATE
___ EOSIN. COUNT

BLOOD BANK

TEST	RESULTS
___ ABO TYPE	
___ Rh TYPE	
___ DIR COOMBS	
___ CORD BLOOD	
___ FETAL SCREEN	
___ RHOGAM WORKUP	

A CANDIDATE FOR RHOGAM

SEROLOGY

TEST	RESULTS	REF. VALUES
___ RPR	______	NON-REACTIVE
___ STREPTOZYME	______	NEGATIVE
___ COLD AGGLUT.	______	NEGATIVE
___ MONO TEST	______	NEGATIVE
___ LE CELL PREP	______	NEGATIVE
___ C-REACT. PROT	______	NONE SEEN
___ RA-LATEX		
___ RUBELLA		
___ FEBRILE PANEL		

MISCELLANEOUS

___ ______
___ ______
___ ______
___ ______
___ ______
___ ______
___ ______
___ ______
___ ______
___ ______
___ ______
___ ______
___ ______
___ ______
___ ______
___ ______
___ ______

74. Mr. Mark C. Zeleski (routine labs)
Hospital number ZM762689
Room 432A
Date: August 5
Physician: M. Hines
Collection times: August 6 AM routine
H&H (hemoglobin and hematocrit)
BMP (basic metabolic profile, chemistry 7)

LABORATORY REQUISITION I

HOSPITAL NO ______________ ROOM NO _____ DATE _________
NAME (LAST) ______________ FIRST ______________ MI ____
ADDRESS ____
PHYSICIAN ____

CHECK SECTIONS ORDERED

___ PROFILES	___ COAGULATION	___ HEMATOLOGY
___ CHEMISTRY	___ URINE TESTS	___ BLOOD BANK
___ SPEC. CHEM.	___ SEROLOGY	___ MISC.

ORDERING INFORMATION

DATE REQUESTED ___/___/___ TIME ORDERED _____ ___ AM ___PM
DATE TO BE DRAWN (IF DIFFERENT THAN ABOVE) ____________
___ ROUTINE ___ASAP
___ STAT ___TIMED __________ ___ AM ___PM

COLLECTION INFORMATION

COLLECTED BY ______________________________
DATE COLLECTED ___/___/___ TIME COLLECTED _____ _____ AM _____ PM
SPECIMEN SOURCE ____ VEIN ____ CAP ____ OTHER (SPECIFY) ____
COMMENTS ______________________________

PROFILES

___ ELECTROLYTES
___ CHEMISTRY 7, METABOLIC
___ CHEMISTRY COMPREHENSIVE
___ CARDIAC PROFILE
___ FOLLOW-UP (8–12 hrs.)
___ FOLLOW-UP (2nd day)
___ LIVER PROFILE
___ THYROID PROFILE
___ LIPID PROFILE
___ GLUCOSE TOLERANCE TEST HRS ___

CHEMISTRY

TEST	RESULTS	RES. VALUES	
___ SODIUM	______	(135-153)	MEQ/L
___ POTASSIUM	______	(3.5-5.3)	MEQ/L
___ CHLORIDE	______	(98-109)	MEQ/L
___ TOTAL CO2	______	(24-31)	MEQ/L
___ GLUCOSE	______	(70-110)	MG/DL
___ BUN	______	(8-23)	MG/DL
___ CREATININE	______	(0.5-1.5)	MG/DL
___ GGTP	______	(7-64)	U/L
___ SGPT (ALT)	______	(10-60)	U/L
___ SGOT (AST)	______	(10-42)	U/L
___ ALK PHOS	______	(26-88)	U/L
___ LDH	______	(91-180)	U/L
___ CPK	______	(22-269)	U/L
___ TRIGLYCERIDES	______	(10-190)	MG/DL
___ CHOLESTEROL	______	(133-240)	MG/DL
___ T-BILIRUBIN	______	(<1.0)	MG/DL
___ URIC ACID	______	(2.5-7.7)	MG/DL
___ PHOSPHORUS	______	(2.5-4.8)	MG/DL
___ CALCIUM	______	(8.5-10.1)	MG/DL
___ TOTAL PROT.	______	(6.0-8.5)	G/DL
___ ALBUMIN	______	(3.5-5.5)	G/DL
___ AMYLASE	______	(44-128)	U/L
___ D-BILIRUBIN	______	(<0.3)	MG/DL
___ CKMB	______	(<5%)	U/L
___ MAGNESIUM	______	(1.6-3.0)	MG/DL
___ ______			
___ ______			
___ ______			

COAGULATION

TEST	RESULTS	REF. VALUES
___ PROTIME (PT)	______	PATIENT SEC.
	______	CONTROL SEC.
___ APTT (PTT)	______	PATIENT SEC.
	______	CONTROL SEC.
___ FIBRINOGEN	______	(200-400) MG/DL
___ FDP	______	(<10) MCG/DL
___ THROMBIN TIME	______	(11-13) SEC.
___ BLEEDING TIME	______	(2.3-9.5) MIN.

URINE TESTS

TEST	RESULTS	REF. VALUES
___ URINALYSIS	______	
___ PREGNANCY TEST	______	
___ CREATININE CLEARANCE	______	M 70-160 ML/MIN F 78-115 ML/MIN
URINE CREAT	______	MG/DL M 1.0-2.0 G/24HR F 0.8-1.8 G/24HR
URINE PROT 24 HOUR	______	(<165) MB/24HR

SPECIAL CHEMISTRY

TEST	RESULTS	REF. VALUES
___ T3 UPTAKE	______	(23-34) %
___ T4	______	(4.5-12.0) UG/DL
___ T7 (FTI)	______	(1.0-4.0)
___ DIGOXIN	______	(0.8-2.0) MG/DL
___ THEOPHYLLINE	______	(10-20) UG/ML
___ PHENYTON	______	(10-20) UG/ML
___ PHENOBARB	______	(15-40) UG/ML
___ GENTAMICIN	______	( ) PK/TR
___ TORBRAMYCIN	______	( ) PK/TR
___ ALCOHOL	______	Toxic > 100 MG/DL
___ CARBAMAZEPHINE	______	(8-12) UG/ML
___ QUINIDINE	______	(2-5) UG/ML
___ NAPA	______	(2-8) UG/ML
___ PROCAINAMIDE	______	(4-8) UG/ML
___ ACETAMINOPHEN	______	(<200) UG/ML
___ LIDOCAINE	______	(1.2-5) MG/ML
___ SALICYLATE	______	(100-200) MG/L
___ LITHIUM	______	(0.5-1.0)
___ DRUG SCREEN	______	SENT TO REF LAB
___ ______		
___ ______		
___ ______		
___ ______		

HEMATOLOGY

___ CBC
___ MANUAL DIFF.
___ HEMOGRAM (Hgb. & Hct.)
___ RETIC. COUNT
___ SED. RATE
___ EOSIN. COUNT

BLOOD BANK

TEST	RESULTS
___ ABO TYPE	
___ Rh TYPE	
___ DIR COOMBS	
___ CORD BLOOD	
___ FETAL SCREEN	
___ RHOGAM WORKUP A CANDIDATE FOR RHOGAM	

SEROLOGY

TEST	RESULTS	REF. VALUES
___ RPR	______	NON-REACTIVE
___ STREPTOZYME	______	NEGATIVE
___ COLD AGGLUT.	______	NEGATIVE
___ MONO TEST	______	NEGATIVE
___ LE CELL PREP	______	NEGATIVE
___ C-REACT. PROT	______	NONE SEEN
___ RA-LATEX		
___ RUBELLA		
___ FEBRILE PANEL		

MISCELLANEOUS

___ ______________________
___ ______________________
___ ______________________
___ ______________________
___ ______________________
___ ______________________
___ ______________________
___ ______________________
___ ______________________
___ ______________________
___ ______________________
___ ______________________
___ ______________________
___ ______________________
___ ______________________
___ ______________________

75. Ms. Anna L. Wojiechowski (Stat Labs)
Hospital number WA938668
Room 435
Date: July 21
Physician: A. Maher
Collection times: July 21 1500
CBC (complete blood count)
Type and Rh

LABORATORY REQUISITION I

HOSPITAL NO ______ ROOM NO ____ DATE ______
NAME (LAST) ______ FIRST ______ MI ____
ADDRESS ______
PHYSICIAN ______

CHECK SECTIONS ORDERED

___ PROFILES ___ COAGULATION ___ HEMATOLOGY
___ CHEMISTRY ___ URINE TESTS ___ BLOOD BANK
___ SPEC. CHEM. ___ SEROLOGY ___ MISC.

ORDERING INFORMATION

DATE REQUESTED ___/___/___ TIME ORDERED ______ ___ AM ___ PM
DATE TO BE DRAWN (IF DIFFERENT THAN ABOVE) ______
___ ROUTINE ___ ASAP
___ STAT ___ TIMED ______ ___ AM ___ PM

COLLECTION INFORMATION

COLLECTED BY ______
DATE COLLECTED ___/___/___ TIME COLLECTED ______ ___ AM ___ PM
SPECIMEN SOURCE ___ VEIN ___ CAP ___ OTHER (SPECIFY) ___
COMMENTS ______

PROFILES

___ ELECTROLYTES
___ CHEMISTRY 7, METABOLIC
___ CHEMISTRY COMPREHENSIVE
___ CARDIAC PROFILE
___ FOLLOW-UP (8–12 hrs.)
___ FOLLOW-UP (2nd day)
___ LIVER PROFILE
___ THYROID PROFILE
___ LIPID PROFILE
___ GLUCOSE TOLERANCE TEST HRS ___

CHEMISTRY

TEST	RESULTS	RES. VALUES	
___ SODIUM	______	(135-153)	MEQ/L
___ POTASSIUM	______	(3.5-5.3)	MEQ/L
___ CHLORIDE	______	(98-109)	MEQ/L
___ TOTAL CO2	______	(24-31)	MEQ/L
___ GLUCOSE	______	(70-110)	MG/DL
___ BUN	______	(8-23)	MG/DL
___ CREATININE	______	(0.5-1.5)	MG/DL
___ GGTP	______	(7-64)	U/L
___ SGPT (ALT)	______	(10-60)	U/L
___ SGOT (AST)	______	(10-42)	U/L
___ ALK PHOS	______	(26-88)	U/L
___ LDH	______	(91-180)	U/L
___ CPK	______	(22-269)	U/L
___ TRIGLYCERIDES	______	(10-190)	MG/DL
___ CHOLESTEROL	______	(133-240)	MG/DL
___ T-BILIRUBIN	______	(<1.0)	MG/DL
___ URIC ACID	______	(2.5-7.7)	MG/DL
___ PHOSPHORUS	______	(2.5-4.8)	MG/DL
___ CALCIUM	______	(8.5-10.1)	MG/DL
___ TOTAL PROT.	______	(6.0-8.5)	G/DL
___ ALBUMIN	______	(3.5-5.5)	G/DL
___ AMYLASE	______	(44-128)	U/L
___ D-BILIRUBIN	______	(<0.3)	MG/DL
___ CKMB	______	(<5%)	U/L
___ MAGNESIUM	______	(1.6-3.0)	MG/DL
___ ______			
___ ______			
___ ______			

COAGULATION

TEST	RESULTS	REF. VALUES
___ PROTIME (PT)	______	PATIENT SEC.
	______	CONTROL SEC.
___ APTT (PTT)	______	PATIENT SEC.
	______	CONTROL SEC.
___ FIBRINOGEN	______	(200-400) MG/DL
___ FDP	______	(<10) MCG/DL
___ THROMBIN TIME	______	(11-13) SEC.
___ BLEEDING TIME	______	(2.3-9.5) MIN.

URINE TESTS

TEST	RESULTS	REF. VALUES
___ URINALYSIS	______	
___ PREGNANCY TEST	______	
___ CREATININE CLEARANCE	______	M 70-160 ML/MIN F 78-115 ML/MIN
URINE CREAT	______	MG/DL M 1.0-2.0 G/24HR F 0.8-1.8 G/24HR
URINE PROT 24 HOUR	______	(<165) MB/24HR

SPECIAL CHEMISTRY

TEST	RESULTS	REF. VALUES
___ T3 UPTAKE	______	(23-34) %
___ T4	______	(4.5-12.0) UG/DL
___ T7 (FTI)	______	(1.0-4.0)
___ DIGOXIN	______	(0.8-2.0) MG/DL
___ THEOPHYLLINE	______	(10-20) UG/ML
___ PHENYTON	______	(10-20) UG/ML
___ PHENOBARB	______	(15-40) UG/ML
___ GENTAMICIN	______	( ) PK/TR
___ TORBRAMYCIN	______	( ) PK/TR
___ ALCOHOL	______	Toxic > 100 MG/DL
___ CARBAMAZEPHINE	______	(8-12) UG/ML
___ QUINIDINE	______	(2-5) UG/ML
___ NAPA	______	(2-8) UG/ML
___ PROCAINAMIDE	______	(4-8) UG/ML
___ ACETAMINOPHEN	______	(<200) UG/ML
___ LIDOCAINE	______	(1.2-5) MG/ML
___ SALICYLATE	______	(100-200) MG/L
___ LITHIUM	______	(0.5-1.0)
___ DRUG SCREEN	______	SENT TO REF LAB
___ ______		
___ ______		
___ ______		
___ ______		

HEMATOLOGY

___ CBC
___ MANUAL DIFF.
___ HEMOGRAM (Hgb. & Hct.)
___ RETIC. COUNT
___ SED. RATE
___ EOSIN. COUNT

BLOOD BANK

TEST	RESULTS
___ ABO TYPE	
___ Rh TYPE	
___ DIR COOMBS	
___ CORD BLOOD	
___ FETAL SCREEN	
___ RHOGAM WORKUP	

A CANDIDATE FOR RHOGAM

SEROLOGY

TEST	RESULTS	REF. VALUES
___ RPR	______	NON-REACTIVE
___ STREPTOZYME	______	NEGATIVE
___ COLD AGGLUT.	______	NEGATIVE
___ MONO TEST	______	NEGATIVE
___ LE CELL PREP	______	NEGATIVE
___ C-REACT. PROT	______	NONE SEEN
___ RA-LATEX		
___ RUBELLA		
___ FEBRILE PANEL		

MISCELLANEOUS

___ ______
___ ______
___ ______
___ ______
___ ______
___ ______
___ ______
___ ______
___ ______
___ ______
___ ______
___ ______
___ ______
___ ______
___ ______
___ ______

CHAPTER 11
Perioperative Care

ACTIVITIES

Vocabulary Exercise

Find the words in the puzzle. If the word is part of a phrase, only the words in italics are hidden in the puzzle. Define each word or phrase.

o	T	M	c	i	r	t	c	e	l	o	c	r	i	C	O
s	U	b	s	c	i	d	e	p	o	h	t	r	o	R	Z
t	m	A	f	r	a	c	t	u	r	e	s	K	l	l	l
e	X	s	H	O	J	r	e	i	n	m	Q	F	p	L	U
o	s	s	i	T	v	N	H	y	d	H	e	e	K	G	S
p	i	u	f	l	M	a	E	p	C	r	r	z	A	t	s
o	s	t	C	M	o	P	C	q	H	i	h	h	n	n	i
r	o	l	J	M	L	b	C	l	o	w	M	M	o	e	s
o	b	u	y	O	w	W	m	p	W	F	v	U	i	m	a
s	m	g	a	A	l	o	e	e	k	W	Z	k	t	t	t
i	o	n	V	d	A	r	S	l	i	Q	k	u	c	r	c
s	r	i	o	z	a	S	x	q	U	t	K	h	u	a	e
d	h	s	d	t	K	a	n	U	B	o	n	h	d	p	l
L	t	A	i	i	u	n	O	Q	J	K	H	a	b	m	e
G	C	v	p	r	o	s	t	h	e	s	i	s	a	o	t
P	e	f	s	n	o	i	t	u	a	c	e	r	p	c	a

1. *abduction* pillow ____
2. *antiembolism* hosiery ____
3. telecasts ____
4. *CircOlectric* bed ____
5. *compartment* syndrome ____

(continues)

6. CPM ______
7. fractures ______
8. ORIF ______
9. orthopedics ______
10. osteoporosis ______
11. PCA ______
12. *perioperative* nursing ______
13. hip *precautions* ______
14. prosthesis ______
15. singultus ______
16. THA ______
17. deep vein *thrombosis* ______

Matching

Match the terms and descriptions.

18. ____ handheld device for respiratory exercises
19. ____ prevents blood clots by massaging the legs
20. ____ halter, belt, or other device used to stabilize injury
21. ____ wire or pin in fractured bone; ropes and weights attached
22. ____ preoperative procedure that requires physician order
23. ____ chemicals that remove hair from skin
24. ____ closed drainage systems
25. ____ excessive blood loss
26. ____ goal of postoperative care
27. ____ contraindications for coughing and deep breathing
28. ____ worn on legs to prevent deep vein thrombosis
29. ____ goal of orthopedic surgery
30. ____ handle with palms of hands
31. ____ monitor the skin at the back of the neck
32. ____ fracture of the upper third or head of the femur
33. ____ care provided before, during, and after surgery
34. ____ provides care while patient recovers from anesthesia
35. ____ inability to expand lungs due to collapse of air sacs

a. depilatories
b. hemorrhage
c. hip fracture
d. graduated compression stockings
e. atelectasis
f. arm sling
g. incentive spirometer
h. keep the fracture in good alignment
i. skeletal traction
j. perioperative care
k. sequential compression therapy
l. postanesthesia care unit
m. shaving the operative site
n. wet cast
o. skin traction
p. eye, nose, rectal, or neurologic surgery
q. Jackson-Pratt and Hemovac
r. early ambulation

Completion

Define the following key reportables when caring for the perioperative orthopedic patient:

36. C ______________________________
37. M ______________________________
38. E ______________________________
39. T ______________________________

Completion

Complete each statement about perioperative care by selecting the proper word from the following list.

1/4 inch	distal	plaster
2 to 4	fanfold	plastic bag
blood clots	fiberglass	pulse oximeter
character	heat	side rail
dangle	hypoxemia	sterile technique
deep breathing	infection control	vital signs
dentures	most common	voiding

40. ______________ ______________ is the primary concern in the operating area.
41. Fingernails should not extend more than ______________ beyond the fingertip.
42. Remove ______________ from a comatose patient to prevent accidental airway obstruction.
43. When making a postoperative bed, ______________ the upper bed linen to the far side of the bed.
44. Take ______________ ______________ upon the patient's arrival to the unit.
45. Check the pulses ______________ to the operative site.
46. Check the ______________ ______________ each time you are in the room.
47. Measure and document the first postoperative ______________.
48. ______________ ______________ coughing clear the air passages.
49. Monitor the amount and ______________ of drainage.
50. Use ______________ ______________ whenever you manipulate or empty a tube or drain or change a dressing.
51. Restlessness, crowing respirations, pounding pulse, and perspiration are signs of ______________.
52. Leg exercises help prevent ______________ ______________.
53. The postoperative patient should ______________ at the bedside for a few minutes before getting up.
54. When the patient is wearing antiembolism hosiery, monitor circulation in the patient's toes every ______________ hours.
55. A ______________ cast dries very rapidly.
56. A ______________ cast may take up to 48 hours to dry completely.
57. The cast gives off ______________ when it dries.
58. Avoid positioning any part of the cast against the ______________ ______________ or footboard.
59. Cover the cast with a ______________ ______________ to enable the patient to shower.
60. The _____ _____ treatment for a fractured hip is a surgical procedure called open reduction internal fixation (ORIF).

Labeling

Label the following diagram.

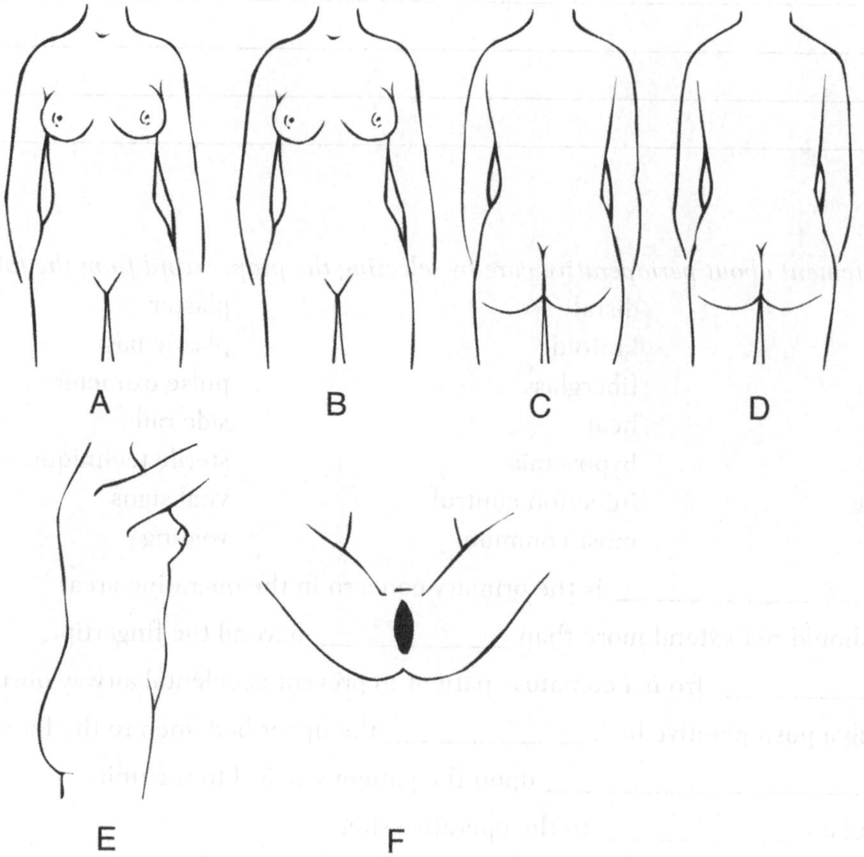

61. Using a colored pencil or crayon, shade in the surgical prep areas that are to be shaved before surgery, as indicated.
    A. abdominal surgery
    B. breast surgery—anterior
    C. breast surgery—posterior
    D. back surgery
    E. kidney surgery
    F. vaginal, rectal, and perineal surgery

Developing Greater Insight

Answer the following questions based on the situation described.

A 75-year-old female patient was admitted to the hospital after low back surgery. Over the first 12 post-operative hours, she received heavy doses of pain medications. At approximately 2:00 a.m., the patient stated that she was cold and requested hot tea. Nursing personnel provided the tea, then left the room. The patient stated that the tea was so hot that she felt as if her lips were burning. In response to the pain, she spilled the hot tea on her chest. She received second- and third-degree burns to her left breast.

The patient sued the hospital and its personnel, contending that their care was substandard in serving a cup of very hot tea to an elderly and heavily medicated patient, then leaving the patient alone and unassisted. The patient also believed the temperature of the tea was so hot that it was unsafe. The patient also claimed that four to six needle procedures would be required to eliminate chronic pain and reduce the scarring that had resulted from her injuries; regardless of those treatments, she would have permanent scarring and disfigurement as a result of her injuries.

62. If a patient requests a cup of hot tea at 2:00 a.m., what action will you take?

____

63. List other methods that could be used to help the patient warm up.

____

64. What method would you use to heat the water for the tea?

____

65. What safety precautions should be taken for an elderly, heavily medicated patient who has a full cup of very hot liquid? _______________

____

The hospital argued that it was not negligent and that the conduct of its nursing staff did not fall below the standard of care. The staff honored the patient's request for hot tea. They stated that when they served the tea, the patient complained it was not hot enough and requested that it be heated further. The staff informed the patient that the tea was hot, and the patient acknowledged the warning.

66. Was it sufficient to warn the patient that the tea was hot? Explain your answer.

____

67. Should the patient have been left alone with the tea? Explain your answer.

____

____

The hospital also disputed the extent of the patient's injuries. They contended that needle injections were not required, and that permanent scarring could have been prevented if the patient had received proper care. The case was settled for $150,000.

68. Review the items listed on the preoperative checklist (page 76). Circle each item for which the PCT is responsible.

Preoperative Checklist

Pt. Name: ______________________________

DOB: ______________________________

O.R. Date: ______________________________

Surgeon: ______________________________

Document	Enclosed?			Information and Follow-Up	Comments
	Yes	No	N/A		
Face sheet	☐	☐	☐		
Consent	☐		☐	Signed and dated by patient, surgeon, and witness. Correct side noted on consent, if applicable.	
H&P	☐	☐	☐	Must be done within 30 days of procedure. Requires an update if done between day 7 and 30.	
Consult, if appropriate	☐	☐	☐		
Old chart, if needed	☐	☐	☐		
ECG done	☐	☐	☐	Required for: Males $\geq$45, females $\geq$50 ☐ Abnormal ECG must be followed up; please comment	
Results available?	☐	☐	☐		
Labs done	☐	☐	☐	☐ Labs pending within 24 hours (comment) ☐ Abnormal labs have been acknowledged ☐ Follow up labs ordered (if applicable) Please make sure to comment in notes.	
Results available?	☐	☐	☐		
Pregnancy test, if applicable	☐	☐	☐	☐ Female $\leq$ age 55 unless hysterectomy or sterilization verified	
Diagnostics	☐	☐	☐	☐ CXR ☐ Stress test ☐ Echo ☐ Cardio consult ☐ Respiratory consult Appropriate tests included and reviewed. Please comment.	
Allergies	☐	☐	☐	Please list all allergies	
Orders	☐	☐	☐	☐ Labs ☐ Bowel prep ☐ ABX ☐ Meds (Allergies noted) ☐ Other	

Document	Enclosed?			Information and Follow-Up		Comments
	Yes	No	N/A			
Meds (home)	☐	☐	☐	Is pt taking: ☐ ASA ☐ Heparin ☐ Coumadin ☐ Other	☐ Continue meds ☐ Hold meds Stop/date: __/__/__	
Daily meds taken with sips of H_2O?	☐	☐	☐			
Preop antibiotics	☐	☐	☐			
Preop meds	☐	☐	☐			
Other meds ordered/given	☐	☐	☐			
Discharge plan	☐	☐	☐	Referral to: ☐ Home Care/Home ☐ Rehab ☐ SNF ☐ Other		
Patient teaching	☐	☐	☐	Please list information that needs to be reinforced.		
Clinical pathway	☐	☐	☐			
Other	☐	☐	☐	Please note:		
NPO Instructions	☐	☐	☐	☐ According to facility policy ☐ Other (please comment)		
NPO since	☐	☐	☐			
Vital signs	☐	☐	☐			
Height	☐	☐	☐			
Weight	☐	☐	☐			
Temperature	☐	☐	☐			
Heart rate	☐	☐	☐			
Respirations	☐	☐	☐			
Blood pressure	☐	☐	☐			
SPO_2 (%)	☐	☐	☐			
O_2 Administration device RA (Room Air)	☐	☐	☐			
Pain scale	☐	☐	☐			
Pt. satisfied	☐	☐	☐			

Document	Enclosed?			Information and Follow-Up	Comments
	Yes	No	N/A		
Quality	☐	☐	☐		
Location	☐	☐	☐		
Pattern	☐	☐	☐		
Sedation scale	☐	☐	☐		
Blood type	☐	☐	☐		
Blood availability- RBC units ___ FFP units___	☐	☐	☐		
Platelet units ___	☐	☐	☐		
Cryo units ___	☐	☐	☐		
Autologous ___	☐	☐	☐		
Glasses/con-tacts removed	☐	☐	☐		
Hearing aids removed	☐	☐	☐		
Dentures removed	☐	☐	☐		
Other prosthe-ses removed	☐	☐	☐		
Device/implant (specify what, where)	☐	☐	☐		
Jewelry removed	☐	☐	☐		
Rings taped?	☐	☐	☐		
Communica-tion barriers?	☐	☐	☐		
Pt prefers to be called ___	☐	☐	☐		
Language spoken ___	☐	☐	☐		
Interpreter ordered	☐	☐	☐		
Contact person name #1	☐	☐	☐		

Document	Enclosed?			Information and Follow-Up	Comments
	Yes	No	N/A		
Relationship	☐	☐	☐		
Contact person name #2	☐	☐	☐		
Relationship	☐	☐	☐		
ID band	☐	☐	☐		
Allergy band	☐	☐	☐		
Blood band	☐	☐	☐		
Preop shower/scrub	☐	☐	☐		
Hair removal	☐	☐	☐	☐ Shave done (physician order required) ☐ Hair clipped ☐ Depilatory ☐ Other (please comment)	
Cap/bath blanket	☐	☐	☐		
TED hose	☐	☐	☐		
Pt has voided (Time) ________	☐	☐	☐		
Bowel prep	☐	☐	☐		
Head up	☐	☐	☐		
Rails up	☐	☐	☐		
Bed in high position	☐	☐	☐		
Operative site/side marked	☐	☐	☐		
By whom: ________	☐	☐	☐		
Anatomic location	☐	☐	☐		
Ambulatory?	☐	☐	☐		
LOC?	☐	☐	☐		

Other information/comments:

Signature & Title:

Date & Time Completed:

Procedural Area Verification and Assessment

Patient Identification (two identifiers):

☐ Name ☐ Date of Birth ☐ Medical Record Number ☐ Social Security Number ☐ Photo ID

Identification Source (one identifier source):

☐ patient statement ☐ parent ☐ guardian ☐ spouse ☐ domestic partner ☐ adult sibling

☐ adult child ☐ facility representative/documents ☐ ID band on

☐ Name/numbers match patient's statement &/or permanent medical record document

Procedure site/side identification

☐ marked ☐ not applicable

Procedure site/side consistent (mark all that apply):

☐ procedure consent ☐ history & physical ☐ physician orders/notes

☐ procedure schedule ☐ diagnostic x-rays/report ☐ marked site

Team members participating in pre-procedure team review and audible verification

☐ anesthesia ______________________ ☐ surgeon ______________________

☐ nurse ______________________ ☐ PCT ______________________

☐ other ______________________ ☐ other ______________________

Signature & Title:

Date & Time Completed:

CHAPTER 12

Heat and Cold Applications

ACTIVITIES

Vocabulary Exercise

Using the definitions provided, unscramble the words.

1. tahueqramia adp ______________________

   A plastic pad with coils on the inside used for heating and cooling
2. tcciornst ______________________

   Make blood vessels smaller
3. ybdo ocre perreutemat ______________________

   The temperature of the deep interior of the body
4. yceparyother ______________________

   Cold treatments
5. midayther ______________________

   Heat treatments
6. edialt ______________________

   Enlarge blood vessels
7. neradlizeeg papicaltino ______________________

   Delivers heat or cold to the entire body
8. thae oxeausthin ______________________

   Condition that develops as a result of overexposure to heat
9. ahet rosket ______________________

   A very serious condition suggesting a profound disruption of the internal mechanisms that control heat in the body
10. yolhrtdrcolao ______________________

    A rectangular tank containing very hot water

11. mahsydrosage ______________________

Using warm, circulating water to relieve pain and muscle spasms, making movement easier

12. yadrothyeraph ______________________

Water therapy

13. yahryiperpex ______________________

Abnormally high body temperature

14. aimytpohher ______________________

Lowering of core body temperature to 95°F or below

15. zocealild piplacaonti ______________________

Delivering heat or cold to a specific area of the body

16. viperetiopera apotherhmyi ______________________

Low body temperature that develops in the operating room

17. aripymr piothmyerha ______________________

Low body temperature that occurs as a result of overwhelming cold stress

18. rasconedy hehrympioat ______________________

Low body temperature that is part of other clinical conditions, such as shock and sepsis

19. zits thab ______________________

A bath in which the pelvic and perineal areas are immersed in warm water; usually done to relieve discomfort following childbirth, perineal, or rectal surgery

20. petdi ______________________

Water that is between 80°F and 93°F

Matching

Match the terms and description.

21.	_____	Often applied immediately after an injury	a. moist hot packs
22.	_____	Applications in which no water touches the skin	b. compresses
23.	_____	Penetrates the tissue to a depth of about 1 centimeter	c. sitz bath
24.	_____	Normal treatment temperature is 105°F	d. dry application
25.	_____	Immersing a body part in 105°F water	e. therapeutic baths
26.	_____	Soaks used for treating small areas	f. aquathermia pad
27.	_____	Small pad through which distilled water flows	g. massage therapy
28.	_____	Packs containing silicate gel in a cotton bag	h. cold therapy
29.	_____	Form of hydrotherapy	i. perioperative hypothermia
30.	_____	Usually given to patients with widespread skin problems	j. eye compresses
31.	_____	Moist, generalized treatment used to reduce fever	k. hot water bottle
32.	_____	Pelvic and perineal areas are immersed in warm water	l. whirlpool
33.	_____	Paper or Styrofoam cups of ice	m. tepid bath
34.	_____	Used for dry, itchy eyes	n. dry heat
35.	_____	Develops in the operating room	o. warm soak

Completion

Complete the table by filling in the terms from the list provided.

aquathermia pad (Aquamatic K-Pad)
cold pack
cool compress
cool soak
disposable (chemical) cold pack
disposable (chemical) warm pack
electric heating pad
gel cold pack
gel warm pack
hot water bottle
hydrocollator pack
hyperthermia blanket
hypothermia blanket
ice bag
ice cap, ice collar
sitz bath
tepid sponge bath
tub bath
warm soak
whirlpool bath

Dry Warm Applications	Dry Cold Applications
36. ______	48. ______
37. ______	49. ______
38. ______	50. ______
39. ______	51. ______

Moist Warm Applications	Moist Cold Applications
40. ______	52. ______
41. ______	53. ______
42. ______	54. ______
43. ______	55. ______
44. ______	56. ______
45. ______	
46. ______	
47. ______	

Write the information in the space provided.

57. Of the items listed in the table (numbers 36 to 56), which is the hottest and most likely to cause injury? ____________________

58. Before using a heat or cold application, you should know the:

 a. ____________________
 b ____________________
 c. ____________________
 d. ____________________
 e. ____________________
 f. ____________________

59. List at least 10 guidelines for giving a whirlpool bath.

 a. ____________________
 b ____________________
 c. ____________________
 d. ____________________
 e. ____________________
 f. ____________________
 g. ____________________
 h. ____________________
 i. ____________________
 j. ____________________

Completion

Complete each statement by selecting the proper word from the following list.

105°F	edema	impaired sensation
115°F	elderly	infants
20 minutes	forearm	paralysis
bleeding	fragile skin	slippery
dry	frostbite	warmed blankets

60. Heat and cold applications are usually not left in place longer than __________, according to the purpose and type of treatment.

61. __________ and __________ patients are very sensitive to heat and cold.

62. Patients with __________, __________, or __________ may be injured by a treatment that is too hot or cold.

63. Sensitive skin begins to burn at about __________, but in some patients this figure could be a little more or less.

64. Prolonged contact with cold may cause __________ and other injuries.

65. Heat should not be used if __________ or __________ is present.

66. With few exceptions, the normal treatment temperature for a heat treatment is __________.

67. Use a thermometer or press the heat application against the inside of your ______________ to check the temperature.

68. Moist heat and cold penetrate much deeper than ______________ applications.

69. Therapeutic bath products may make the tub ______________.

70. ______________ may increase comfort for elderly patients.

Developing Greater Insight

Answer the following questions based on the situation described.

A 34-year-old female patient was admitted from a local nursing home for care of urosepsis from a urinary catheter infection. The patient was a paraplegic from an auto accident, and had resided in various nursing homes for a decade. Despite the paralysis, the patient complained of pain and regularly took oral medications for pain relief. She apparently complained of pain and a cold sensation in her feet. A staff person applied hydrocollator packs to the feet and the patient sustained serious burns. There was no proper physician order for the hydrocollator packs, and most of the personnel on the unit were not familiar with their use. Very few personnel on this unit were approved for and qualified to apply hydrocollator hot packs to patients. The patient stated that the hydrocollator packs were uncovered when they were applied to her feet. The injury was not reported to other nursing personnel or the physician. When the feet were examined, the patient was found to have multiple second- and third-degree burns. They were debrided and treated, and skin grafting was done. However, after several years the patient had not healed properly and continued to be at risk of amputation of both legs below the knee. The facility was sued and settled for an undisclosed seven-figure amount. As a result of this incident, one nurse's license was revoked, and another nurse was disciplined by the licensure board.

71. If a patient complains of pain and having cold feet, what actions can the PCT take?

____

72. What safety precautions will you take when applying hydrocollator packs to a patient?

____

73. Were hydrocollator packs contraindicated in this paralyzed patient?

____

74. What should you do if you are instructed to apply a hydrocollator pack and no prefitted cover is available?

____

75. Assuming that you are instructed to apply a hydrocollator pack, how often will you check the patient's skin under the pack?

____

76. What signs and symptoms of burns would you look for under a hydrocollator pack?

____

77. If you suspect that a patient is being burned by a heat treatment, what action will you take?

____

78. Is a physician order needed for hydrocollator packs to be applied to a patient's feet?

____

79. What is the maximum length of time for hydrocollator packs to be applied?

____

CHAPTER 13

Caring for Patients with Special Needs

ACTIVITIES

Vocabulary Exercise

1.–22. Fill in the words in the puzzle using the clues and definitions provided.

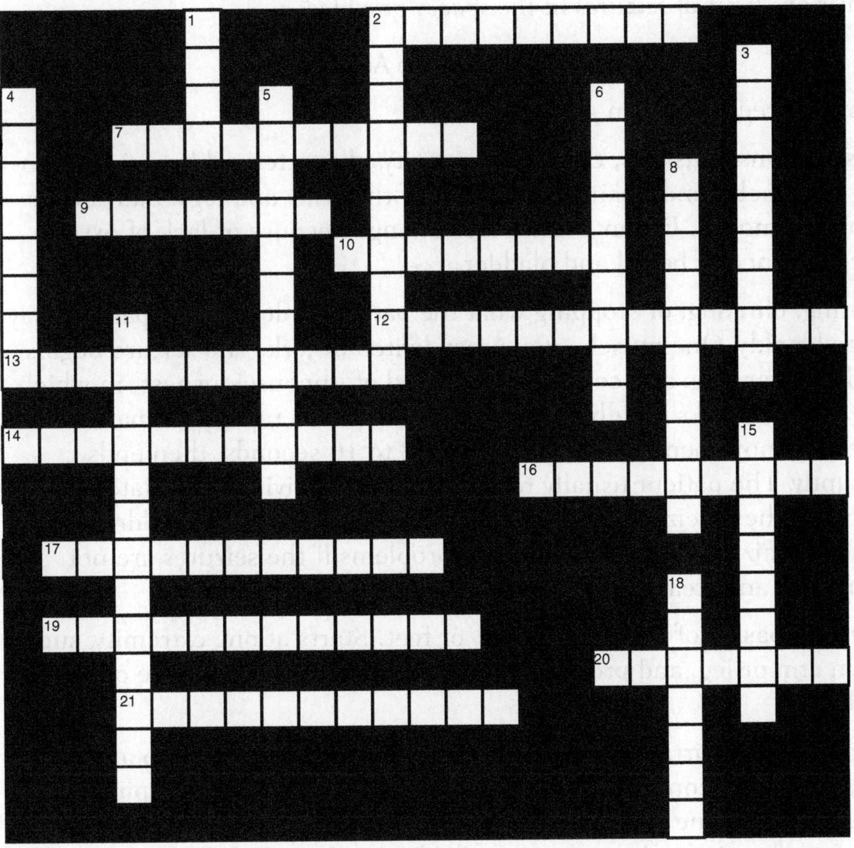

ACROSS

2. Loss of movement and impairment of various parts of the body.
7. To worsen or make worse.
9. A sudden, spontaneous episode of excessive and scrambled electrical activity caused by interference with impulses in the brain.
10. An acute confusional state caused by reversible medical problems; common in elderly persons.
12. A treatment in which various biologic agents are given to alter the patient's immune response to eliminate cancer.
13. Autonomic _____ is a potentially life-threatening complication of spinal cord injury that indicates uncontrolled sympathetic nervous system activity.
14. Seizure _____ are individualized measures that keep the patient safe during an unexpected seizure.
16. _____ therapy involves the use of high-energy, ionizing beams to the site of the cancer.

(continues)

17. A communication professional who mediates between speakers of different languages.
19. The use of medications or drugs to destroy cancer.
20. Patients with _____ paralysis experience loss of muscle tone and absence of tendon reflexes.
21. An ancient practice that involves placing tiny, thin needles in various parts of the body to correct imbalances in energy.

DOWN

1. A sensation, vision, smell, taste, or bright light that signals the onset of a seizure.
2. Paralysis of the lower half of the body, including both legs; bowel and bladder control are also lost.
3. The period of time immediately after a seizure.
4. _____ woman syndrome is similar to posttraumatic stress disorder, and is seen in people threatened with death or serious injury in extremely stressful situations.
5. Paralysis affecting the arms and legs.
6. A small instrument that measures the radiation dose to which each individual is exposed when working with the patient.
8. _____ disorders are medical conditions present at birth.
11. A form of radiation therapy in which tiny radioactive seeds or pellets are implanted directly inside the body.
15. Domestic _____ is a pattern of forced behaviors that may include repeated battering and injury, psychological abuse, sexual assault, progressive social isolation, deprivation, and intimidation.
18. In _____ paralysis, the extremities move in an involuntary pattern, similar to muscle spasms.

Completion

Complete the table by identifying the various types of seizures in the spaces provided.

Type of Seizure	Signs of Seizure Activity
23. _______________	May be preceded by an aura. Loss of consciousness, convulsive activity, characterized by rigid stiffening of muscles and jerking movement of the arms and legs. Saliva runs from the mouth. Patient's color may change because of lack of oxygen. Incontinence of bowel and bladder.
24. _______________	Staring, blinking, or stopping what the patient is doing. The patient may stare blankly. One muscle group may twitch or jerk. The seizure begins without warning, and consists of a period of unconsciousness, in which the patient blinks rapidly, stares blankly, breathes rapidly, or makes chewing movements. The seizure lasts 2 to 10 seconds, then ends abruptly. The patient usually resumes normal activity immediately. Because these seizures are mild, they may go unnoticed. Children with absence seizures may have learning problems if the seizures are not identified and treated.
25. _______________	Muscle spasms of the face, hands, or feet. Starts at one extremity, such as an arm or leg, and progressively moves upward on that side of the body.
26. _______________	Abnormal acts, irrational behavior, or loss of judgment due to a temporary change in consciousness. Automatic behavior, such as typing or eating, may continue normally. The patient may uncontrollably smack the lips, wander aimlessly, or uncontrollably twitch part of the body.
27. _______________	Consists of one or more myoclonic jerks. The patient remains conscious but cannot control the muscle movement.

Type of Seizure	Signs of Seizure Activity
28. ________________	Multiple seizures occurring simultaneously with no break between seizures. When this seizure begins, the patient cries out, then falls to the floor. The muscles stiffen (tonic phase), then the extremities begin to jerk and twitch (clonic phase). The patient may lose bladder control. Consciousness returns slowly. After this seizure, the patient may feel tired, or be confused and disoriented. This state may last from a few minutes to several hours or days. The patient may fall asleep, or gradually become less confused until full consciousness returns.

True/False

Circle T if the statement is true or F if it is false.

29. T F Status epilepticus is a seizure that lasts for a long time, or repeats without recovery.
30. T F A person can have a seizure without actively convulsing.
31. T F Seizure prevention is the PCT's primary concern when caring for patients who have seizure disorder.
32. T F The patient who is on seizure precautions may safely be left alone in the tub for five minutes.
33. T F Always take an oral temperature on patients who are on seizure precautions.
34. T F Patients swallow their tongues when having a seizure.
35. T F After a seizure, the patient may be drowsy, confused, and require periodic reorientation.
36. T F Chemotherapy drugs cannot differentiate cancer cells from normal cells, so they destroy some healthy cells.
37. T F Pressure ulcers are the most common cause of autonomic dysreflexia.
38. T F Patients with alopecia have hair loss.
39. T F Chemotherapy is not excreted from the body.
40. T F Problems that seem minor can trigger autonomic dysreflexia.
41. T F Treatment for autonomic dysreflexia involves rapidly identifying the condition and giving strong medications to lower blood pressure.
42. T F Patients with leukemia are at high risk of infection.
43. T F Radiation therapy destroys cancerous tissue without damaging healthy tissue.
44. T F Brachytherapy is a form of chemotherapy in which tiny medicated seeds or pellets are implanted directly inside the body.
45. T F A radiation symbol is blue or black with an orange background.
46. T F Side effects of immunotherapy usually cease within a week after beginning treatment.
47. T F Rehabilitation is a skilled service provided by licensed therapists.
48. T F The nursing assessment data are the most accurate indicators of the existence and intensity of pain.
49. T F Constipation is a common side effect of pain medication, and goes away over time.
50. T F Patients with implantable medication pumps are at risk of meningitis and other brain infections.

51. T F Check with the RN before sending the patient who has an implantable medication pump for an MRI.

52. T F Use a transfer belt when moving a postoperative patient with a newly implanted medication pump.

53. T F Permanent leg numbness and weakness are normal for patients who have epidural catheters.

54. T F Pain has no effect on the length of recovery in individuals with acute illness.

55. T F The RN is responsible for monitoring each patient's bowel activity carefully and documenting it on the flow sheet.

56. T F Restorative nursing complements skilled rehabilitation.

Completion

Complete the following tables in the spaces provided.

Principle of Rehabilitation and Restoration	Description
57. ______________________	Starting restorative care early in the disease or admission will improve the outcome.
58. ______________________	Keep the patient as active as possible, considering his or her medical condition. Encourage patients to be as independent as possible. For example, giving passive range-of-motion exercises prevents deformities and complications. However, active range-of-motion exercises done by the patient will prevent deformities and strengthen muscles.
59. ______________________	Follow the care plan to prevent injury and deformity. Practice safety.
60. ______________________	Emphasizing what the patient can do gives the patient confidence and provides hope. Instead of saying, "You cannot use your right arm," say, "You can use your left arm."
61. ______________________	You have learned that you cannot isolate the medical problem from the rest of the person. Consider all of the patient's strengths and needs. Use and build on the strengths to overcome the needs. Communicate strengths, so others can use them to help the patient as well.

Type of Pain	Description
62. ______________________	Occurs suddenly and without warning. Is usually the result of tissue damage, caused by conditions such as injury or surgery. Typically decreases over time, as healing takes place.
63. Persistent (chronic) pain	______________________________

Type of Pain	Description
64. ______________________	Occurs as a result of an amputation. For example, the patient who has had a leg removed complains of pain in the toes. The pain is real, not imaginary.
65. Radiating pain	______________________

Labeling

Mrs. Torres has a cerebral thrombus. Follow the maze to identify its location.

66. *Use your knowledge of medical terminology to identify the body part affected by defining the following words.*

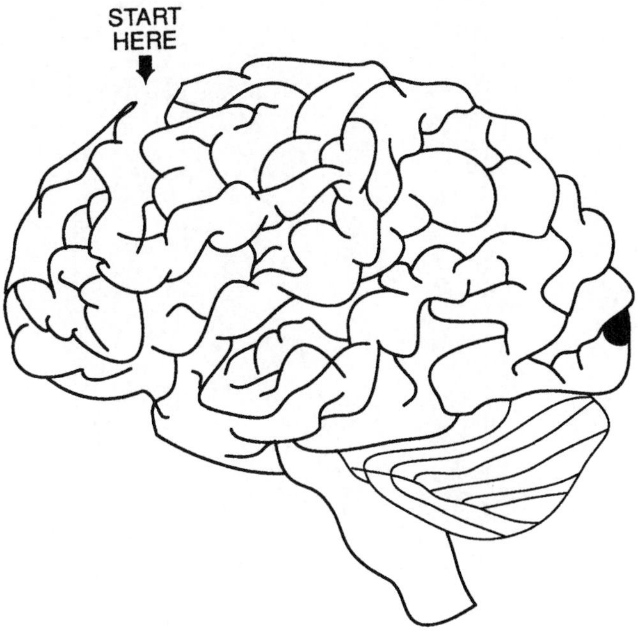

67. Cerebral ______________________

68. Thrombus ______________________

Developing Greater Insight

Answer the following questions based on the situation described.

A patient contended that he had agonizing postoperative pain after surgery, which he described as like being "on fire." The patient and his wife testified they requested help at least five times. The following day, a nurse discovered that the epidural line was broken or disconnected, so the patient had not been receiving his postoperative pain medication. The patient claimed that the period of prolonged pain caused him great emotional distress, and that he still experiences nightmares. The hospital admitted that the epidural catheter had been disconnected at some point within a two-hour time frame, but denied negligence. Nursing notes revealed that personnel checked the line regularly, and that it was intact. The hospital contended that the epidural catheter, which was very small, became dislodged due to patient movement. They claimed it had been disconnected for only a brief time, and that personnel had administered other medications to relieve the pain during this period. The hospital sent the patient a letter apologizing for the problems he encountered during his hospital stay. The jury returned a verdict for the defense, and nothing was awarded to the patient.

69. What nursing actions can you take to help a patient who is having pain? ____

70. When a patient has an external catheter leading to the spine, what actions can you take to prevent it from becoming dislodged? ____

71. How did documentation help this hospital staff? What can you learn from this? ____

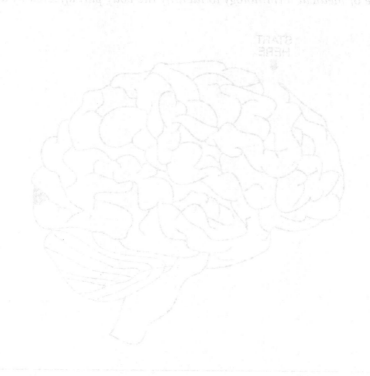

CHAPTER 14
Respiratory Procedures

ACTIVITIES

Vocabulary Exercise

1.–21. Fill in the words in the puzzle using the clues and definitions provided.

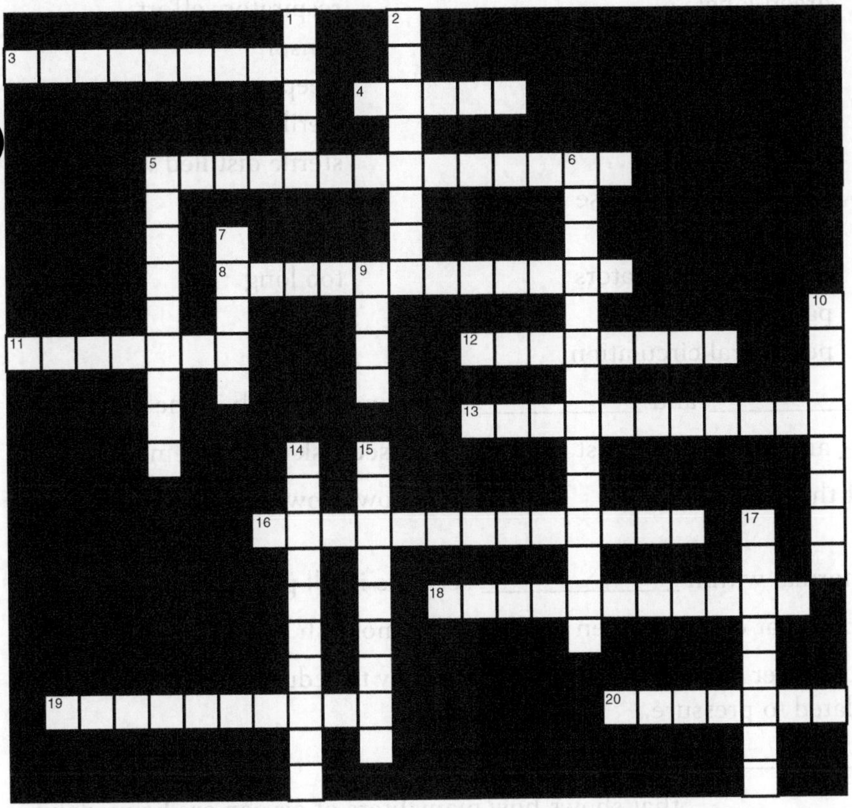

ACROSS

3. A condition in which there is insufficient oxygen in the blood.
4. _____ maintains positive airway pressure during both inspiration and expiration.
5. The _____ mask is used to deliver oxygen to patients with severe hypoxemia. It has one-way plastic flaps on the sides through which the patient's exhalations can escape, but outside air cannot enter. A reservoir bag is connected to the bottom of the mask.
8. Oxygen is a _____ item.
11. The lungs give off carbon _____, a waste product.
12. Sleepiness for no apparent reason.
13. The air _____ mask mixes oxygen with room air to obtain the percentage of oxygen ordered by the physician.
16. An _____ airway is most commonly used to keep the airway open in unconscious patients.
18. When the patient has _____, the chest appears to sink in just below the neck, and/or under the breastbone or rib cage, with each inhalation in an effort to take more air into the lungs.
19. A water bottle that moistens the oxygen for comfort and prevents drying of the mucous membranes in the nose, mouth, and lungs.
20. A small tube for oxygen administration with two prongs that fit into the patient's nostrils.

(continues)

DOWN

1. The pressure _____ is connected to the flow meter on an oxygen cylinder, and shows how much oxygen is in the cylinder.
2. The pulse _____ is an instrument that measures the level of saturation of the patient's hemoglobin with oxygen.
5. An inhalation dispenser that converts liquid medicine into a mist that can be inhaled by the patient.
6. A _____ airway is a curved, soft rubber device that is inserted through one nostril, and may be used in responsive patients.
7. Patients with sleep _____ may stop breathing hundreds of times a night, then snore loudly when they start to breathe again.
9. The _____ device holds the airway open and maintains positive pressure in the chest throughout the respiratory cycle.
10. _____ drainage technique uses gravity to help drain and remove secretions from the lungs; commonly used in the care of patients with cystic fibrosis.
14. Cupping the hands and clapping against the patient's chest wall to loosen secretions.
15. _____ refill is an indication of the patient's peripheral circulation and shows how well the tissues are being nourished with oxygen.
17. A rigid plastic suction called a "tonsil tip."

Completion

Complete each statement by selecting the proper word from the following list.

10	flow meter	replace
2–3	green label	respiratory effort
5	head of the bed	sensor
5 liters	hemoglobin	sleep apnea
500	humidifier	sterile
absorb	immobile	sterile distilled water
acid	Legionnaire's disease	stimulated
anticoagulant	modify	tongue
carbon dioxide	oxygen concentrators	too long
cough	patient	
face	peripheral circulation	

22. Death will result if levels of _____________ and _____________ become too high in the body.
23. Patients who are _____________ and those on bedrest have an increased risk of hypoxemia.
24. Capillary refill is an indication of the patient's _____________ and shows how well the tissues are being nourished with oxygen.
25. Capillary refill should return to normal within _____________ seconds in all patients.
26. _____________ is the part of blood that carries oxygen to the cells to nourish them.
27. Rotate the position of the pulse oximeter clip _____________ regularly to reduce the risk of skin breakdown and complications related to pressure.
28. Oxygen is color-coded with a _____________ in the United States.
29. Oxygen flow is regulated by a _____________ that shows how many liters of oxygen are being delivered to the patient each minute.
30. Most facilities consider oxygen cylinders empty when the pressure reaches _____________ pounds.
31. A _____________ is usually attached to the oxygen administration equipment if the patient's liter flow exceeds _____________ liters.
32. Fill the oxygen humidifier with _____________.

33. Inhalation of tap water is associated with an increased incidence of _____________.

34. An oxygen mask should not be used with liter flows under _____________ because it may cause rebreathing of the patient's exhaled carbon dioxide, and has a smothering effect.

35. Elevate the _____________ when the patient is receiving oxygen.

36. The patient's gown and bed linen _____________ extra oxygen from the air.

37. _____________ cannot deliver flows over 5 liters.

38. The most common cause of airway obstruction is the _____________.

39. Do not try to _____________ the oral airway if the patient removes it or spits it out.

40. The nasopharyngeal airway should not be used for patients receiving _____________ medications.

41. If the patient gags or coughs after you have inserted the nasopharyngeal airway, the airway may be _____________.

42. Suction for no more than _____________ seconds at a time, including the time it takes to withdraw the catheter.

43. A nerve in the airway may be _____________ by the suction catheter, altering the pulse rate.

44. Suction catheters are _____________.

45. Always monitor the _____________ and not the equipment.

46. Never _____________ the oxygen equipment to make it fit together.

47. After a nebulizer treatment, encourage the patient to _____________

48. The cardinal sign of _____________ is excessive daytime sleepiness.

49. The CPAP mask must fit tightly against the _____________.

50. The BiPAP device cycles in response to the patient's _____________.

Completion

Complete the table in the spaces provided.

Pulse Oximeter Value	Interpretation/Meaning
95% to 100%	51.
86% to 90%	52.
71% to 85%	53.
Below 75%	54.

Labeling

Label the following diagrams.

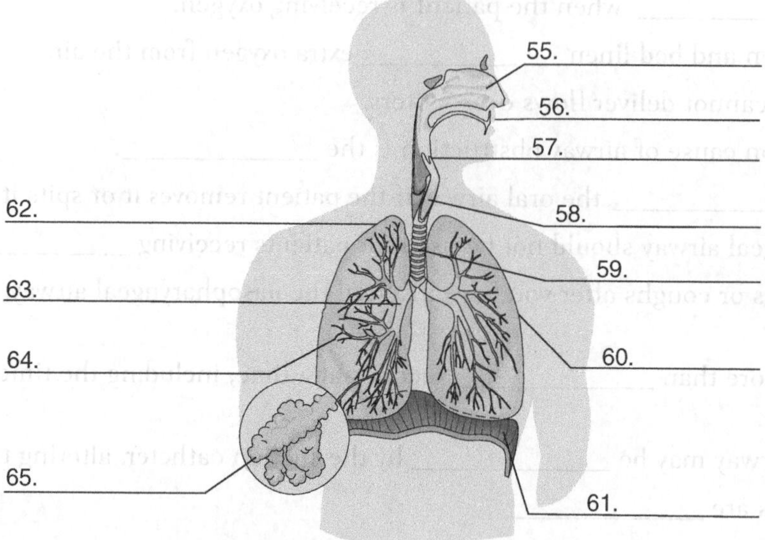

55. ______________________________

56. ______________________________

57. ______________________________

58. ______________________________

59. ______________________________

60. ______________________________

61. ______________________________

62. ______________________________

63. ______________________________

64. ______________________________

65. ______________________________

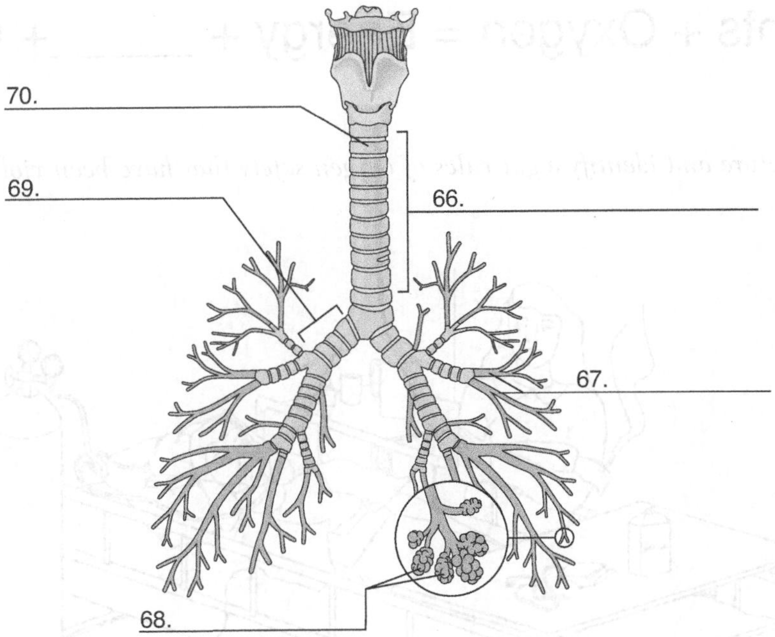

66. ______

67. ______

68. ______

69. ______

70. ______

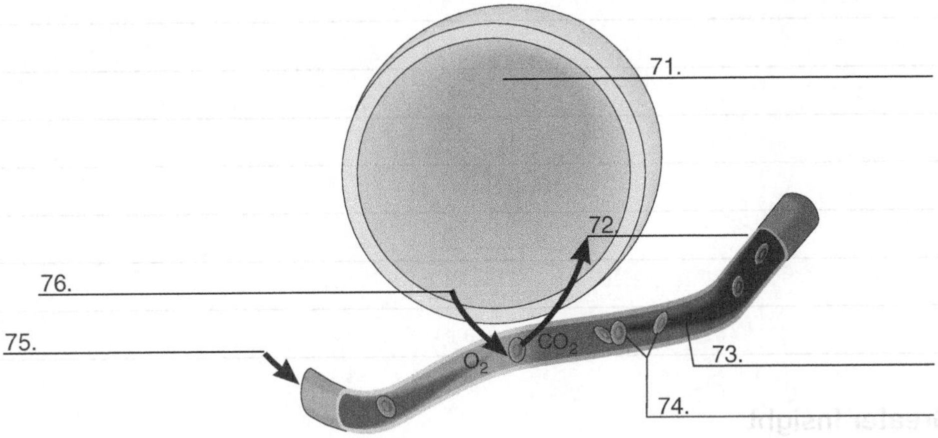

71. ______

72. ______

73. ______

74. ______

75. ______

76. ______

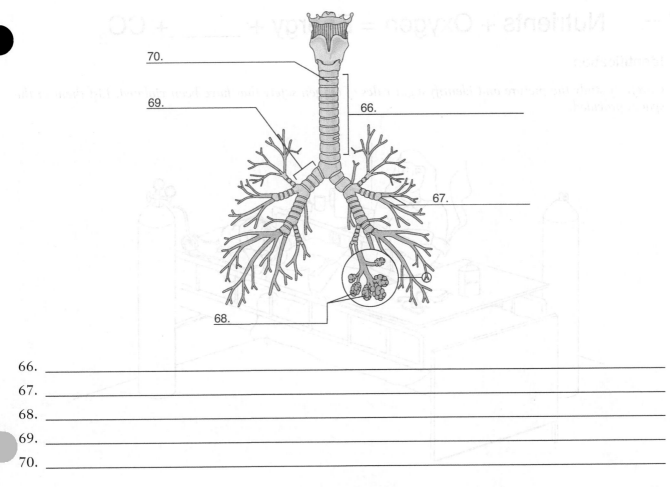

77. Nutrients + Oxygen = Energy + ______ + CO_2

Identification

Carefully study the picture and identify eight rules of oxygen safety that have been violated. List them in the spaces provided.

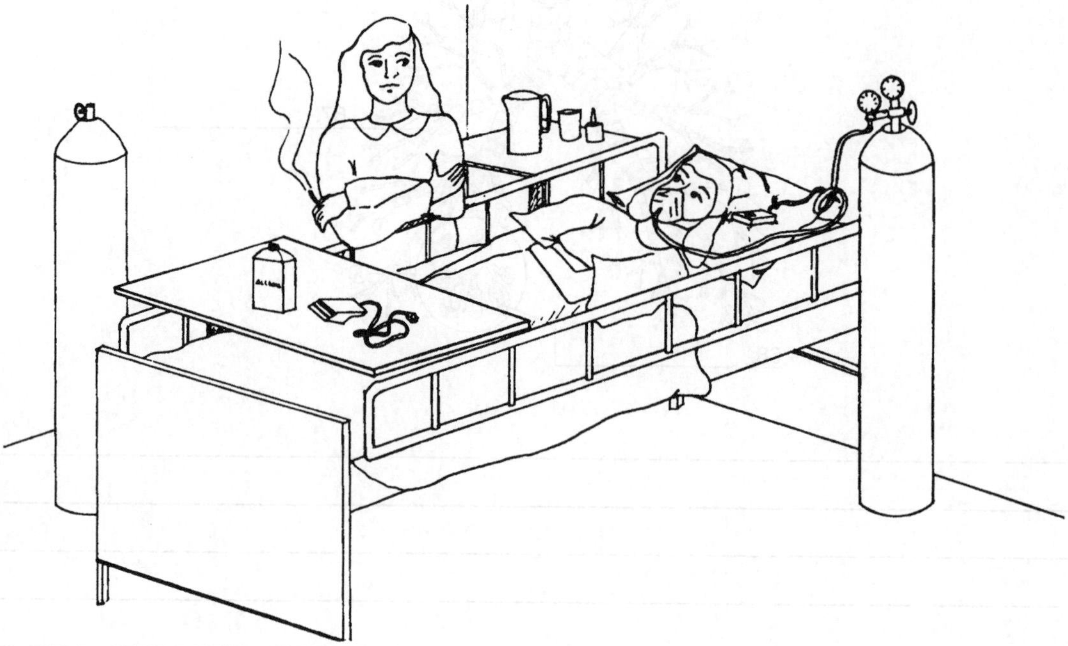

78. ______________________________
79. ______________________________
80. ______________________________
81. ______________________________
82. ______________________________
83. ______________________________
84. ______________________________
85. ______________________________

Developing Greater Insight

Answer the following questions based on the situation described.

A 63-year-old female patient was admitted to the hospital and diagnosed with pneumonia. The patient's condition deteriorated at some point after her transfer from the emergency room to a seventh-floor bed. The family contended that over the next three hours, the unit was short of personnel and failed to follow physician orders to monitor the patient's oxygen level carefully. The patient sustained hypoxemia and was close to respiratory arrest when her condition was identified and treated. She was left with permanent brain damage affecting her physical and mental abilities. She understands most information, but cannot talk, and requires 24-hour care.

86. What are signs and symptoms of hypoxemia that may be seen in a patient with pneumonia?

____

____

____

____

87. How often should a newly admitted patient whose condition is not known to you, who is using oxygen by mask, be monitored? ____

____

The family claimed that the patient would be in normal physical health today if the unit had not been understaffed and personnel had monitored the pulse oximeter and notified the physician regarding critical changes in the patient's condition. Family members produced hospital documents and testimony from current and former employees showing that the hospital purposely understaffed to increase profits, which increased the risk of injury to patients. The hospital denied negligent staffing, stating that there was a severe nursing shortage in the community.

88. What pulse oximeter values would you expect to see for a patient who is in respiratory distress?

____

89. What pulse oximeter values would you expect to see for a patient who has a life-threatening emergency?

____

This case was settled for $2.7 million six days before trial, but the settlement required the family to sign a confidentiality agreement. The family had wanted to tell the story to the news media, hoping to pressure the hospital into correcting problems and thereby prevent harm to future patients. The family refused to settle unless the confidentiality clause was removed. The hospital removed the confidentiality clause a few days before trial, and the patient's story was well covered by television news and made the front page of many local newspapers.

CHAPTER 15
Advanced Respiratory Procedures

ACTIVITIES

Vocabulary Exercise

1.–17. *Fill in the words in the puzzle using the clues and definitions provided.*

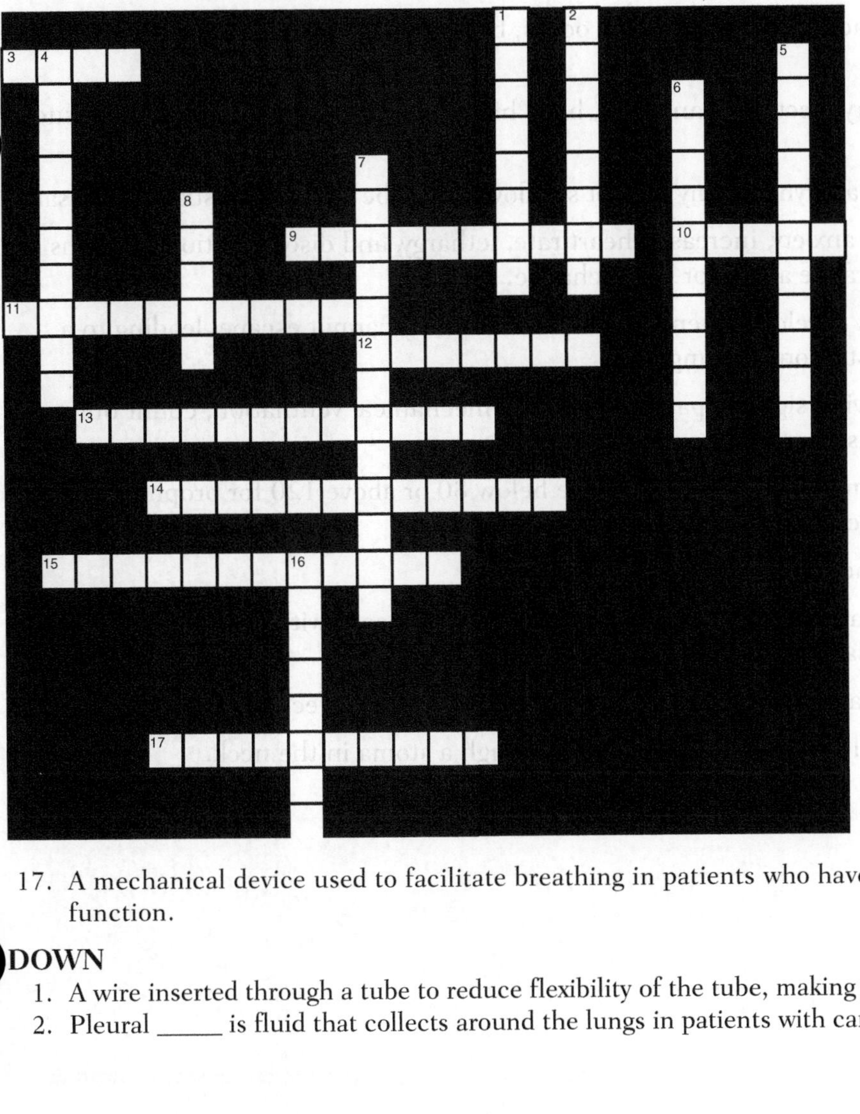

ACROSS

3. Twill _____ are often used to hold the tracheostomy apparatus in place at the neck.
9. Enlargement of abdomen caused by air taken in during resuscitation.
10. Chest _____ are sterile, plastic tubes that are inserted through the skin of the chest, between the ribs and into the space between the pleural membrane that covers the lung and the pleural membrane that lines the chest wall.
11. Suction catheters are measured in _____.
12. The plastic outer (or inner) tube for a tracheotomy.
13. Surgical removal of the larynx.
14. Free air in the chest cavity outside the lung.
15. The instrument used to perform the intubation procedure.
17. A mechanical device used to facilitate breathing in patients who have impaired respiratory or diaphragm function.

DOWN

1. A wire inserted through a tube to reduce flexibility of the tube, making insertion easier.
2. Pleural _____ is fluid that collects around the lungs in patients with cancer.

(continues)

4. Endotracheal _____ is a measure that provides complete control over the airway.
5. A surgical procedure to create an opening into the neck through which to breathe.
6. Blood in the chest cavity.
7. Before the patient is intubated, he or she is well oxygenated by using a bag-valve mask _____.
8. The external opening on the skin surface of a tracheotomy.
16. The _____ position gets its name because the patient appears to be smelling a flower or other object.

True/False

Circle T if the statement is true or F if it is false.

18. T F To remove the inner tracheostomy cannula, turn the adapter at the end clockwise.
19. T F When ventilating a patient who has an endotracheal tube or tracheostomy, squeeze the bag once every 5 to 8 seconds, or as directed.
20. T F Caring for a new tracheostomy is a sterile procedure.
21. T F Ventilate against the patient's breathing rhythm with the bag-valve mask, as this will stimulate spontaneous ventilations.
22. T F Insert the tracheostomy dressing with the split facing down.
23. T F Do not remove the old tracheostomy ties until the new ties are in place.
24. T F When the larynx is removed, there is no connection between the upper and lower airways.
25. T F A patient who has a tracheostomy can smell odors, blow his or her nose, and suck on a straw.
26. T F A patient who has a laryngectomy can smell, blow his or her nose, whistle, gargle, and suck on a straw.
27. T F A patient who has had a laryngectomy cannot swallow, so a tube feeding is usually necessary.
28. T F Restlessness, dyspnea, anxiety, increased heart rate, lethargy, and disorientation are signs of ineffective airway clearance and poor gas exchange.
29. T F Tension pneumothorax develops when air in the chest cavity cannot escape, leading to a steady buildup of pressure on the lung.
30. T F When monitoring the vital signs of patients who use mechanical ventilation, count only ventilator-delivered breaths.
31. T F Pressures in the suction machine should not be below 80 or above 120 for oropharyngeal and nasopharyngeal suctioning.
32. T F Hemothorax occurs when there is blood in the lungs.
33. T F If a glass chest tube drainage bottle accidentally breaks, replace it with a spare plastic drainage bottle immediately.
34. T F Patients who are mechanically ventilated are at very high risk of infection.
35. T F The patient can control expulsion of secretions through a stoma in the neck.

Labeling

Label the following diagrams.

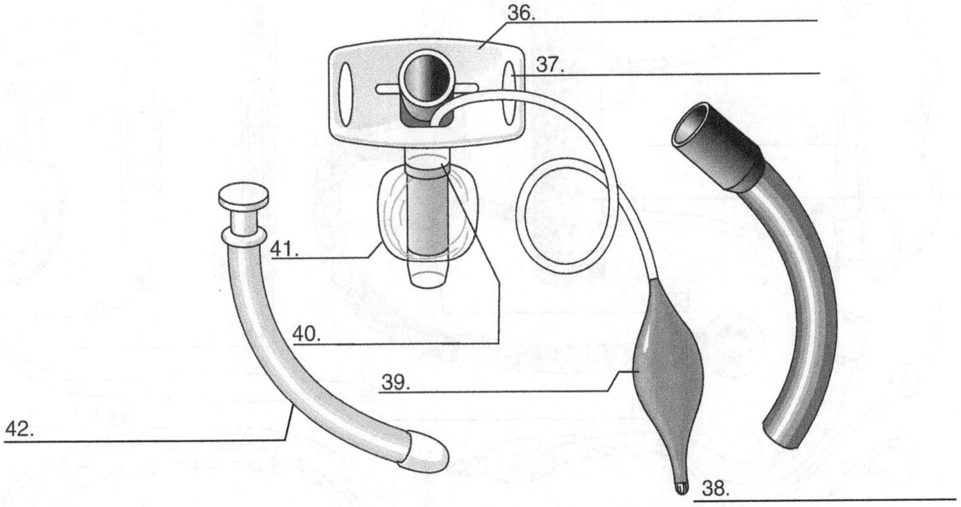

36. ____
37. ____
38. ____
39. ____
40. ____
41. ____
42. ____

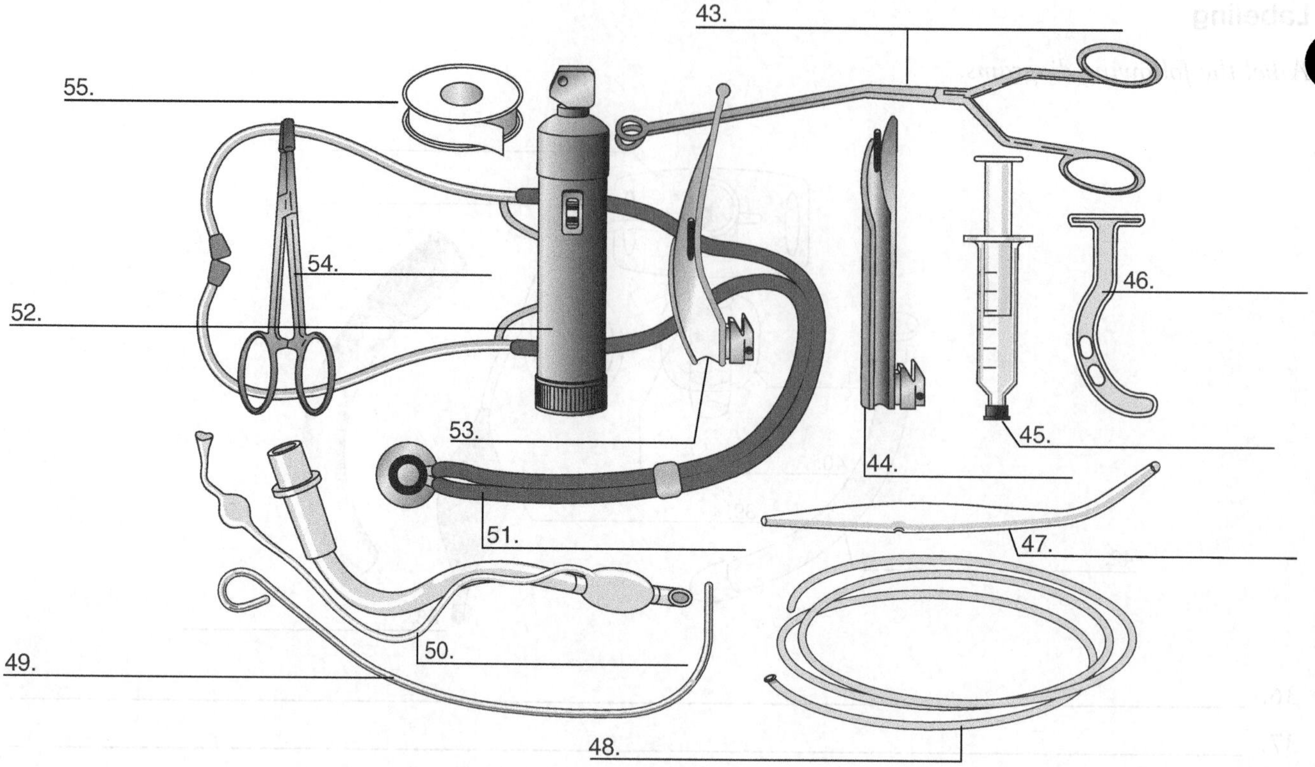

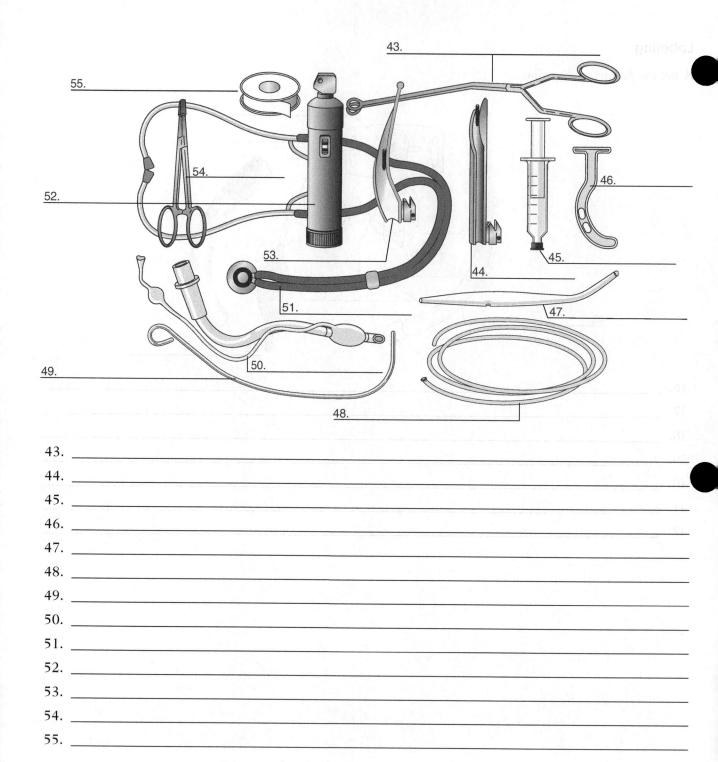

43. ______________________________
44. ______________________________
45. ______________________________
46. ______________________________
47. ______________________________
48. ______________________________
49. ______________________________
50. ______________________________
51. ______________________________
52. ______________________________
53. ______________________________
54. ______________________________
55. ______________________________

Developing Greater Insight

Answer the following questions based on the situation described.

A 54-year-old patient was admitted to the hospital's intensive care unit with diagnoses of pneumonia and renal failure. He was intubated and placed on a ventilator. The tube became plugged with secretions and the patient experienced respiratory arrest. The staff called a code and the patient was resuscitated. The patient and his wife sued the hospital, alleging that the personnel failed to properly monitor the patient and evaluate his condition, and failed to recognize that the tube was blocked. They further alleged that staff failed to call a physician and failed to immediately call a code when the emergency was first noted. The patient experienced cardiac arrest before being resuscitated. He is permanently brain-damaged, in a persistent semi-vegetative state, and is fed through a PEG tube. He will require lifetime care.

56. What are signs and symptoms that an endotracheal tube has to be suctioned?

____

____

____

57. What types of things would a PCT monitor in a patient who uses an endotracheal tube connected to a ventilator? ____

____

____

58. What signs and symptoms would you expect to see if a patient was in respiratory distress?

____

____

____

The patient and his wife sued for lost income, past and future medical expenses, and pain and suffering. Prior to this event, the patient earned $50,000 per year as a computer technician. The plaintiff estimated future medical costs of $4 million; the defense determined that the cost of lifetime care would be $1.5 million. A jury found in favor of the patient and awarded a negligence judgment plus expenses, for a total of $5,152,416.

CHAPTER 16
Cardiac Care Skills

ACTIVITIES

Vocabulary Exercise

1.–35. *Fill in the words in the puzzle using the clues and definitions provided.*

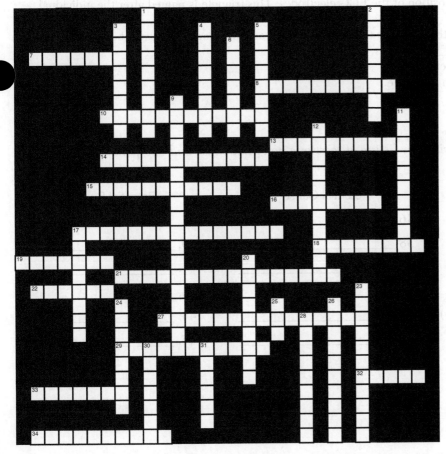

ACROSS

7. Leads I, II, and III are standard or _____ leads.
8. When a patient has _____ PVCs, several irritable sites within the ventricles act as pacemakers.
10. Ventricular _____ is a form of cardiac arrest.
13. A myocardial _____ is a heart attack.
14. High blood pressure.
15. An _____ is an X-ray study of the blood vessels.
16. The AV node may also be called the _____.
17. A condition that means the person is likely to develop high blood pressure in the future.
18. The resting phase of the heart cycle.
19. Palpate the _____ pulse in the groin.
21. The _____ node is located on the bottom of the atrium, just above the ventricles.
22. Contrast _____ is a special dye that is injected through the blood vessels so they can be seen during certain X-ray procedures.
27. Cardiac _____ is a diagnostic procedure in which a catheter is threaded through the blood vessels into the heart.

(continues)

29. An abnormal heart rhythm.
32. The cardiac ___ consists of a working and a resting phase.
33. An instrument that amplifies sounds, similar to a stethoscope.
34. The lower chambers of the heart.

DOWN

1. _____ monitoring enables the patient to be ambulatory.
2. _____ PVCs mean the pacemaker is coming from one irritable area within the ventricles.
3. The _____ pedis pulse is in the foot.
4. The central _____ is a reference system at the intersection of leads I, II, and III.
5. An abnormal rhythm in which every other heartbeat is a PVC.
6. The difference between the apical pulse and radial pulse is the pulse _____.
9. The cardiac monitor and _____ measure electrical activity within the heart and display the information on a screen.
11. The normal pacemaker to the heart is the _____ node.
12. Rapid heart rate.
17. The electrical impulse travels through the right and left bundle branches and _____ fibers.
20. A rhythm in which a PVC appears every third beat.
23. During the _____ phase of the heart cycle, the heart beats, pumping blood to the body.
24. In _____ monitoring, the patient's heart rhythm is displayed on a monitor at the bedside, and at another remote location, usually the nurses' station.
25. After the electrical impulse leaves the upper heart, it travels downward through a network of fibers, called the bundle of _____.
26. The _____'s triangle displays the position of the ECG electrodes. This triangle is named after the individual who invented the ECG.
28. The electrical signals reflected in the leads are tiny and far away from the heart. They must be enlarged by the ECG machine, and are called _____ limb leads.
30. The working phase of the heart cycle.
31. Check the posterior _____ pulse in the ankle.

Completion

Complete the table in the spaces provided by listing at least one potential cause and one potential solution for each problem.

Problem	Potential Cause	Potential Solution
Wandering baseline	36. _____	37. _____
Skin irritation from electrodes	38. _____	39. _____
False alarm—low rate	40. _____	41. _____
False alarm—high rate	42. _____	43. _____
60-cycle interference (baseline fuzzy)	44. _____	45. _____
Artifact	46. _____	47. _____
Low amplitude	48. _____	49. _____

Completion

Complete the table in the spaces provided by identifying the number of pacemaker impulses from each area of the heart.

	Area of the Heart	Pacemaker Rate
50.	______________________	20–40
51.	AV node	______________________
52.	______________________	60–100

Labeling

Using the following figure, label the areas of the heart and electrical impulses transmitted from each.

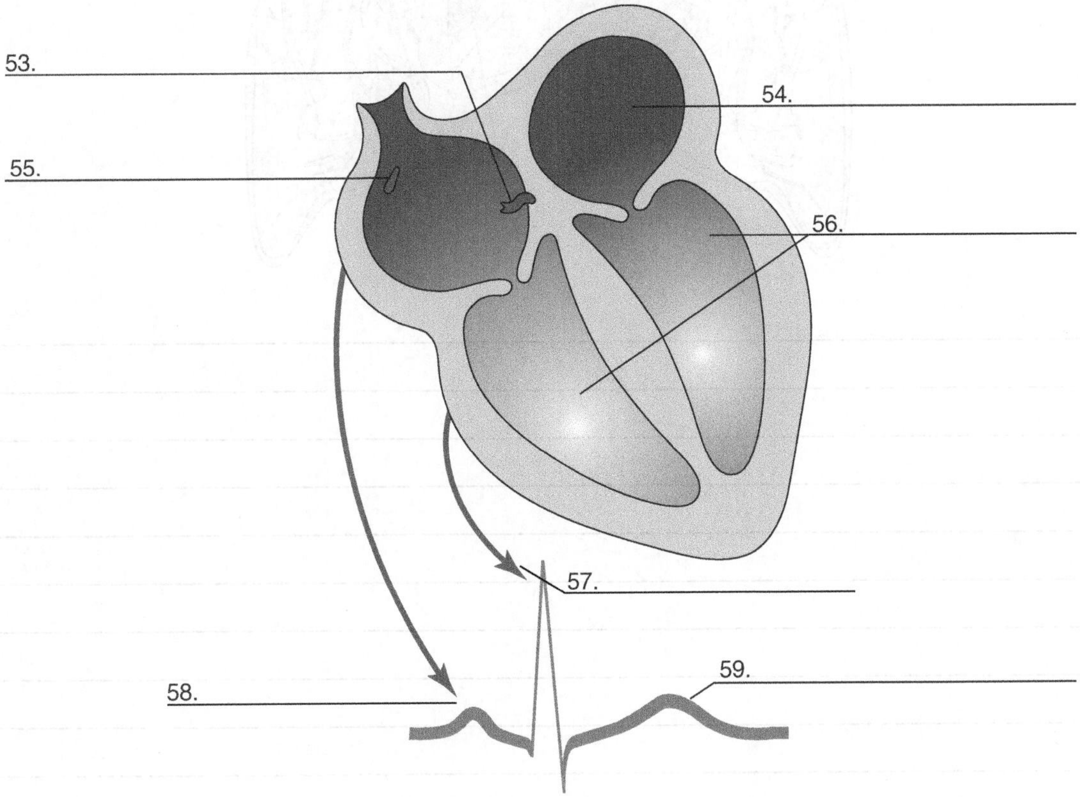

53. ______________________
54. ______________________
55. ______________________
56. ______________________
57. ______________________
58. ______________________
59. ______________________

Trace the flow of blood from the heart to the lungs, then back to the heart. Use a red-colored pencil to trace the path of freshly oxygenated blood, and a blue-colored pencil to trace the path of deoxygenated blood. Label each area.

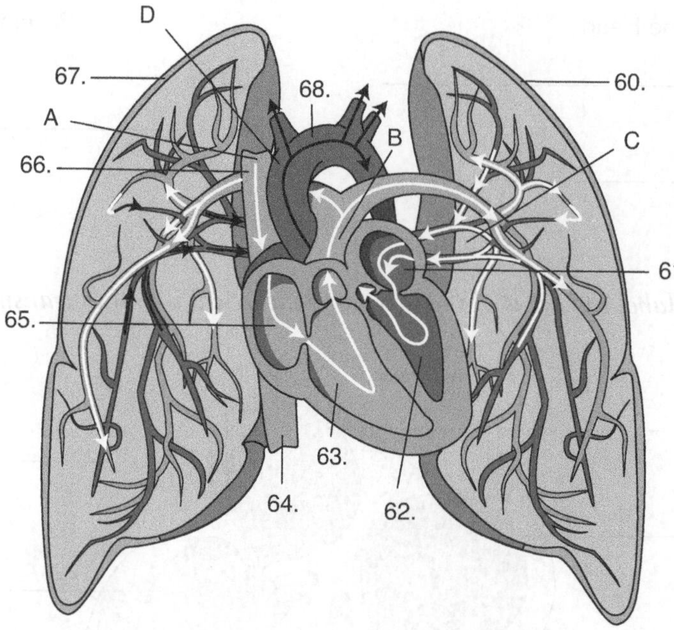

60. ______________________________

61. ______________________________

62. ______________________________

63. ______________________________

64. ______________________________

65. ______________________________

66. ______________________________

67. ______________________________

68. ______________________________

A. ______________________________

B. ______________________________

C. ______________________________

D. ______________________________

Identification

Identify 10 pulses in the body.

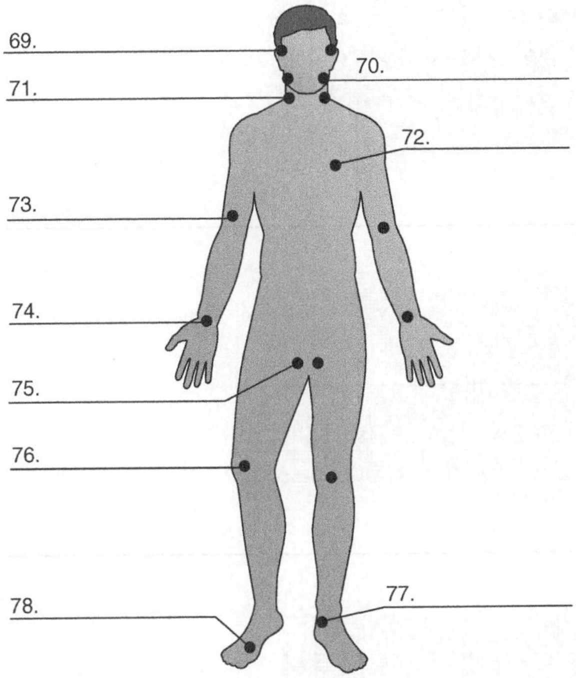

69. ______________________________
70. ______________________________
71. ______________________________
72. ______________________________
73. ______________________________
74. ______________________________
75. ______________________________
76. ______________________________
77. ______________________________
78. ______________________________

Identify the cardiac rhythms in the diagrams.

79. 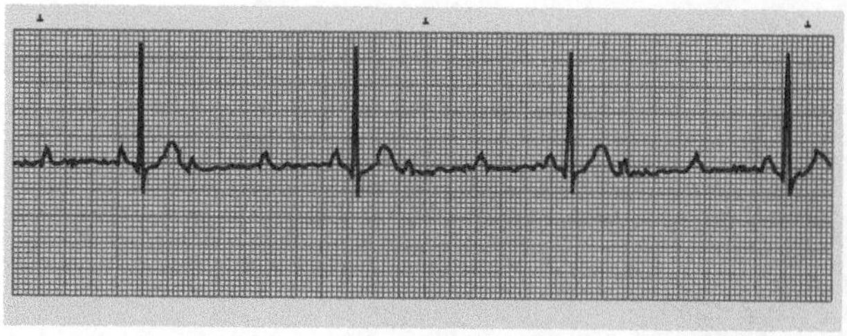

____

80. 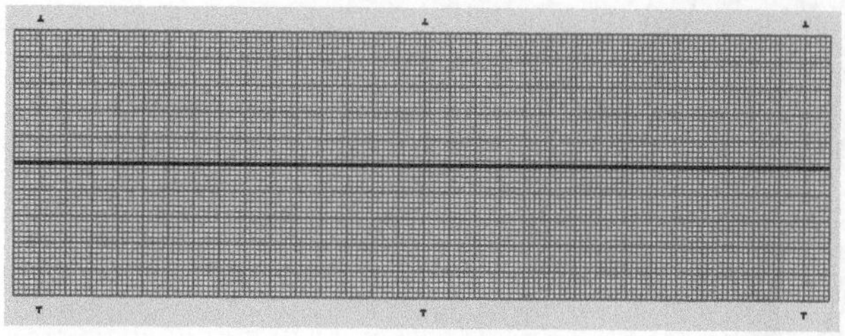

____

81. 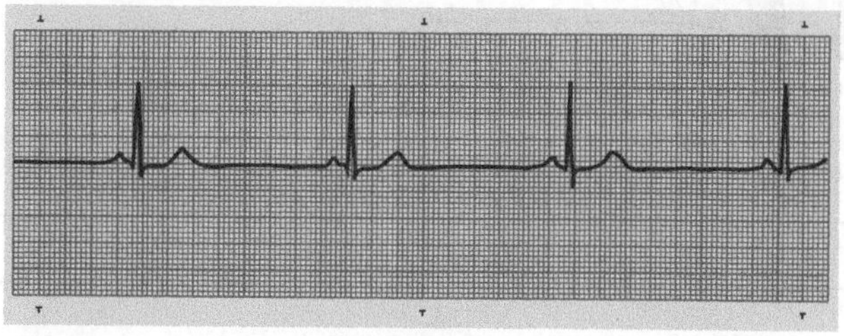

____

82. 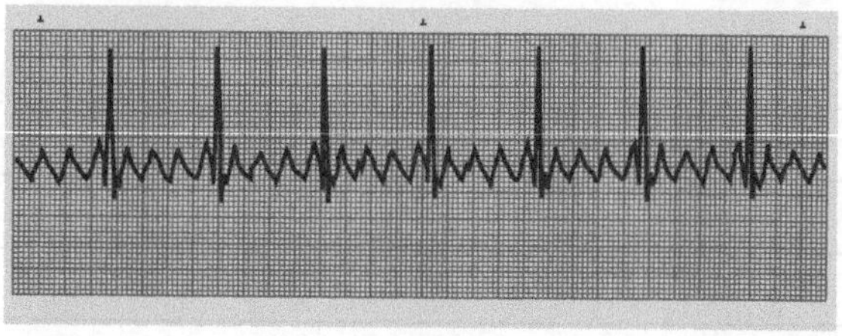

____

83. 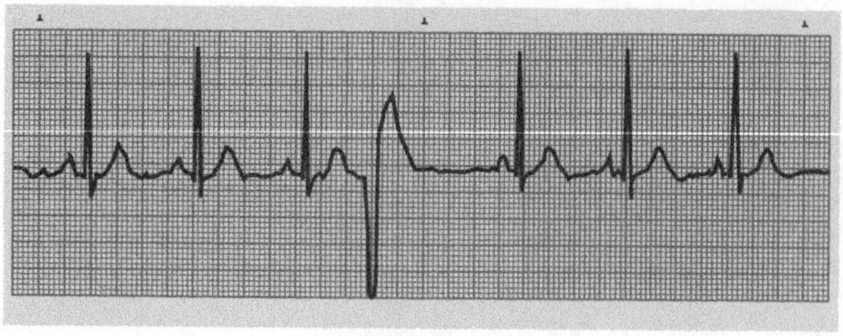

____

84. 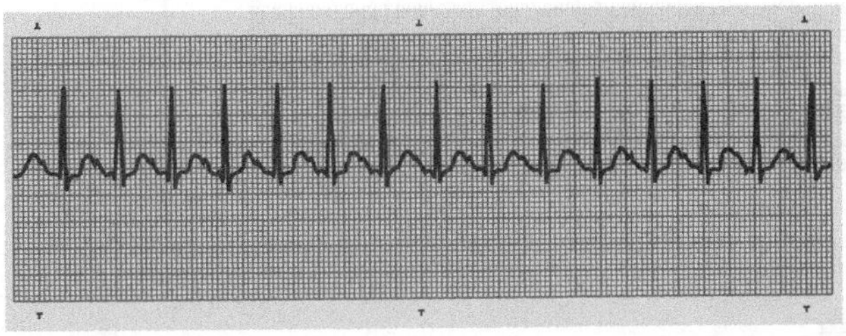

85. 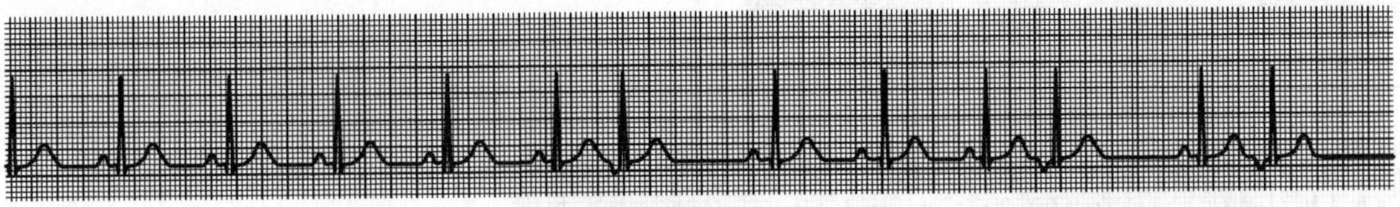

86. 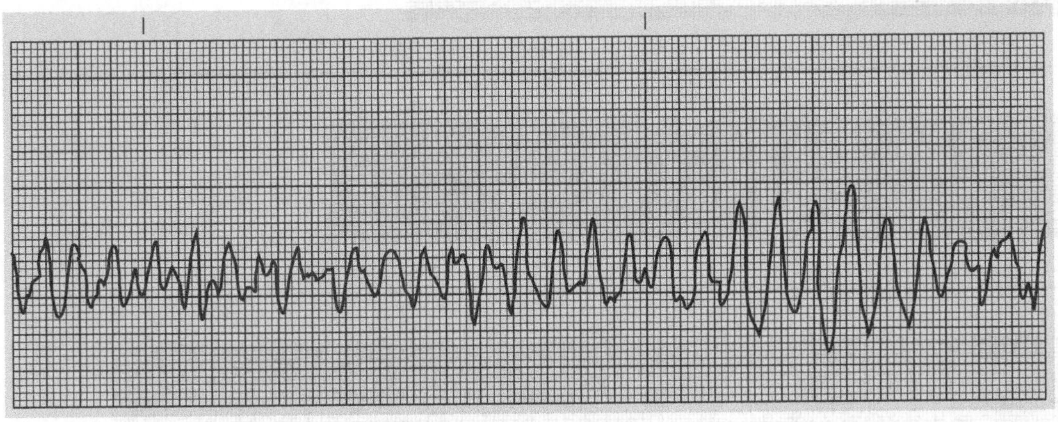

87. 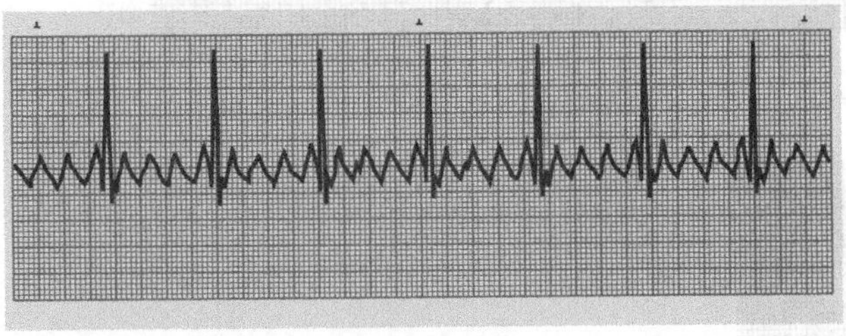

88. 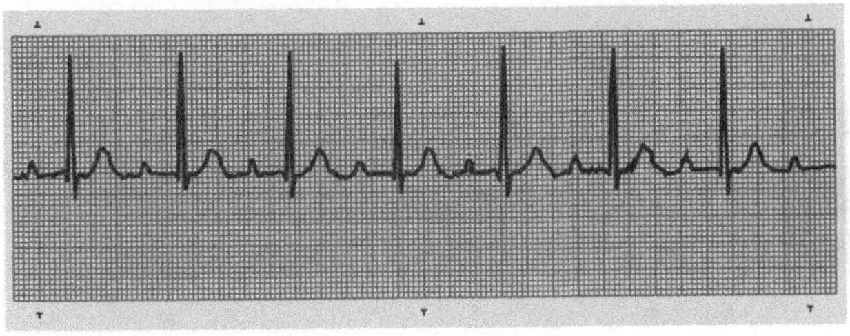

89. 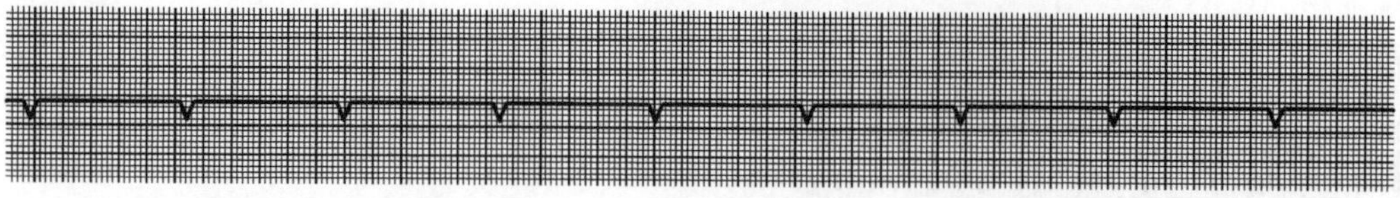

90. 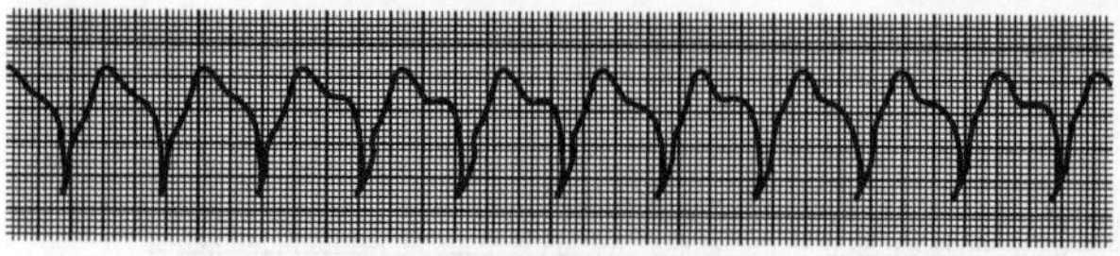

91. 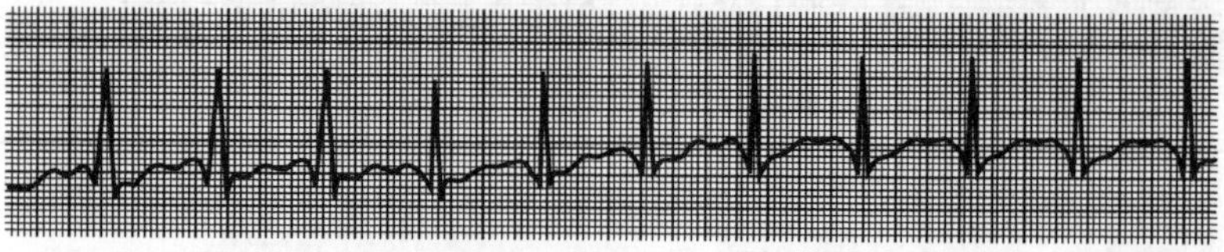

92. 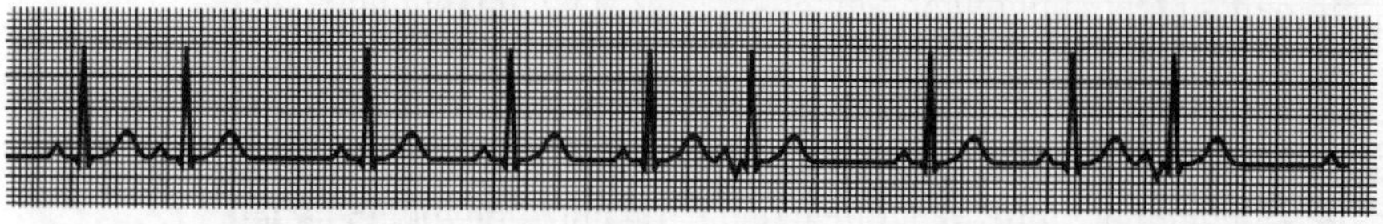

93. 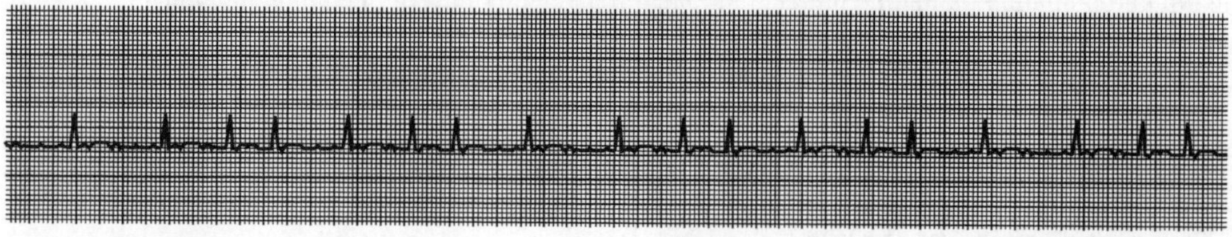

94. 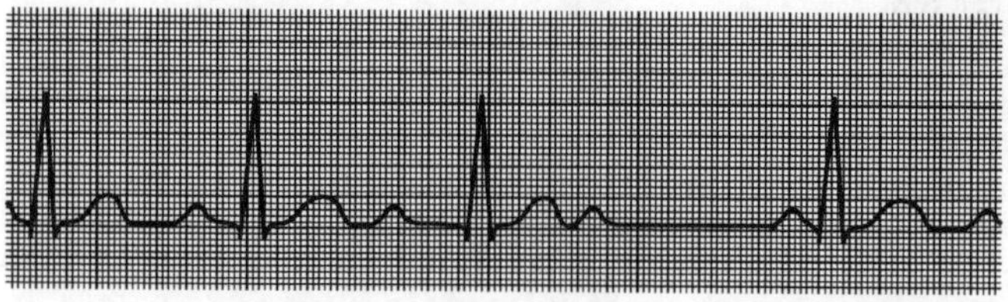

95. 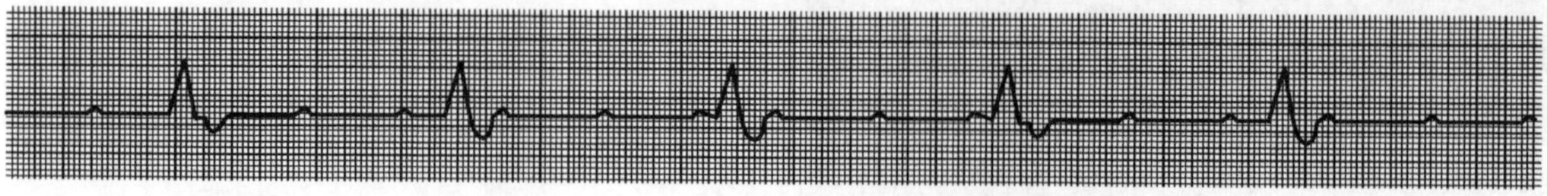

96. 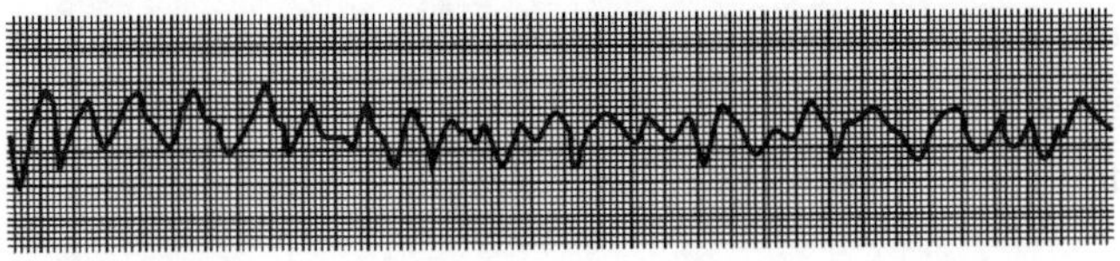

____

97. 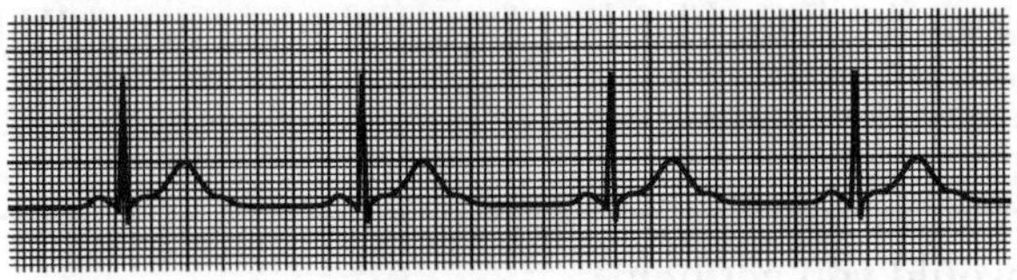

____

98. 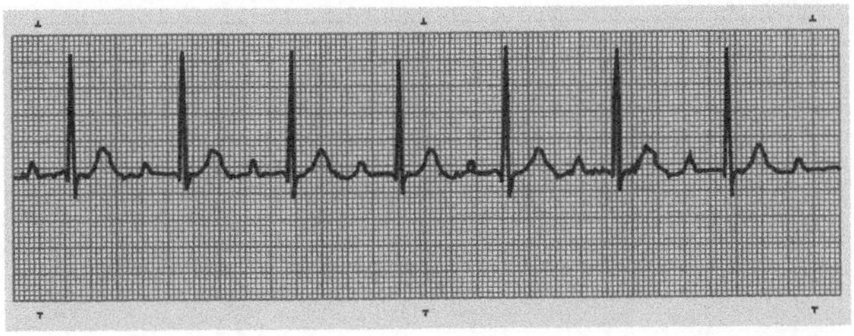

____

99. 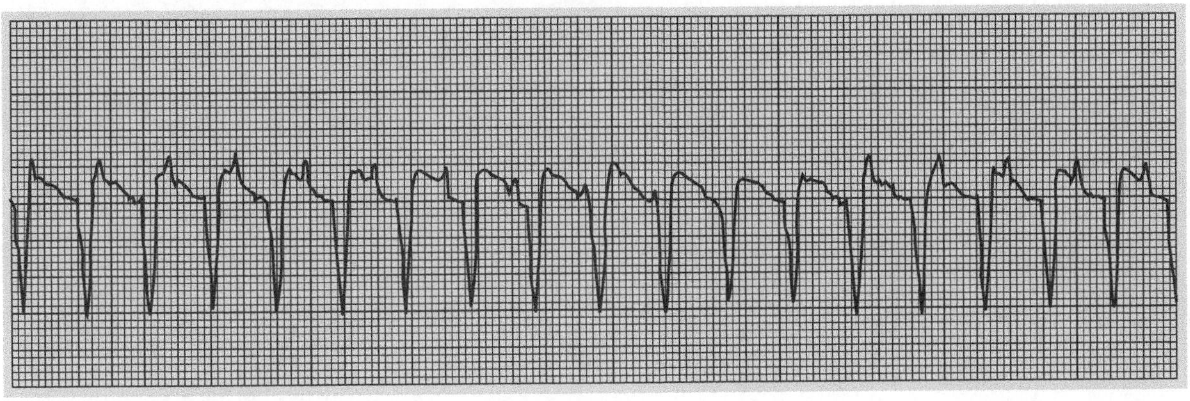

____

Developing Greater Insight

Answer the following questions based on the situation described.

A 72-year-old patient was hospitalized for surgical revision of a perforated duodenal ulcer. After surgery, the patient was admitted to the intensive care unit for 10 days. On day 10, she was transferred to the telemetry unit. The patient died within eight hours of being admitted to the telemetry unit. The record reveals that the nurse saw the patient in bed at 12:30 a.m. At 1:05 a.m., staff found the patient unresponsive in a pool of blood on the floor of her room. Her central venous catheter was disconnected. Personnel called a code, but the patient could not be resuscitated. The cause of death was listed as hemorrhage. The patient's family contended that the hospital was negligent in supervising the patient. They noted that the patient was being continuously monitored by telemetry, and that an alarm would sound if the patient's heart rate was abnormal. The telemetry system was in good working order. The family stated that the failure of staff to respond to the alarms contributed to the patient's death; if not for their negligence, she would be alive today. The hospital disagreed with the allegations of negligence.

It said the patient was in poor health and would not have lived long. The case settled out of court with a payment of $125,000 to the patient's family.

100. Should staff respond to the patient's room each time a telemetry alarm sounds? Why or why not?

____

____

101. What action would you take if you found a patient on the floor bleeding from a disconnected IV line?

____

____

102. If you found a patient on the floor bleeding, how would you get help?

____

____

CHAPTER 17
Emergency Procedures

ACTIVITIES

Vocabulary Exercise

Find the words in the following puzzle. If the word is part of a phrase, only the words in italics are hidden in the puzzle. Define each word or phrase.

c	t	r	a	l	u	c	i	r	t	n	e	v	c	d
e	h	s	r	e	c	o	v	e	r	y	M	a	e	e
n	n	o	e	A	E	D	M	E	I	n	i	f	l	j
d	t	o	k	r	t	k	r	G	O	d	i	b	m	a
o	G	j	i	i	r	W	i	z	r	b	a	c	a	i
t	T	e	U	t	n	a	T	a	r	r	T	r	n	m
r	Z	A	H	Y	a	g	c	i	u	j	M	a	e	r
a	r	T	w	t	R	t	l	d	F	E	E	s	u	e
c	a	p	M	F	t	l	i	f	s	L	F	h	v	h
h	e	n	A	e	a	a	v	c	a	c	q	M	e	t
e	l	v	k	t	i	w	C	G	s	i	O	x	r	o
a	c	c	i	r	P	u	x	U	j	u	l	m	A	p
l	o	o	w	m	r	P	T	x	H	b	s	u	V	y
p	n	a	t	h	r	u	s	t	K	H	g	e	r	h
b	y	a	d	j	u	n	c	t	i	v	e	F	r	e

1. *adjunctive* airway device ______________________
2. AED ______________________
3. airway ______________________
4. respiratory *arrest* ______________________
5. *cardiac* arrest ______________________

(continues)

6. choking ______________________
7. clear ______________________
8. *crash* cart ______________________
9. defibrillation ______________________
10. *durable* power of attorney for health care ______________________
11. *endotracheal* tube ______________________
12. respiratory *failure* ______________________
13. hypothermia ______________________
14. head-tilt, chin-lift *maneuver* ______________________
15. *pocket* mask ______________________
16. *recovery* position ______________________
17. resuscitation ______________________
18. jaw-*thrust* maneuver ______________________
19. *ventricular* fibrillation ______________________

Identification

Identify the meaning of each of the following abbreviations:

A
B
C

20. A = ______________________
21. B = ______________________
22. C = ______________________

C
P
R

23. C = ______________________
24. P = ______________________
25. R = ______________________

Completion

Complete the following statements by filling in the terms from the list provided.

1/4	crash cart	six
1/3	four	speak
3	immediately	spine
12	jaw-thrust maneuver	stand back
15	lips	sternum
20	living will	supine
21	newborn infant	tongue
asystole	oral airway	upside down
bag-valve mask	pocket mask	ventricular fibrillation
breathe	postresuscitation care	vital
cough	replace	

26. After ____________ to ____________ minutes without oxygen, the patient's brain begins to die.
27. Resuscitation is most successful if performed ____________.
28. During CPR, the heart is squeezed between the ____________ and the ____________.
29. CPR is approximately 1/4 to ____________ as effective as the normal heartbeat.
30. The most common cause of airway obstruction is the ____________ falling into the back of the throat.
31. Cold exposure preserves the ____________ organs.
32. The normal respiratory rate in adults is ____________ to ____________ respirations per minute.
33. Opening the airway is most effective when the patient is lying in the ____________ position.
34. Use only the ____________ to open the airway of patients who have known or suspected neck injuries.
35. A patient will be unable to ____________, ____________, or ____________ with a complete airway obstruction.
36. When assisting the patient to breathe using an adjunctive device, connect an oxygen source and run the oxygen at ____________ liters per minute, or as high as possible.
37. Room air contains approximately ____________ percent oxygen.
38. Monitoring the color of the patient's ____________ will help you see how well the patient is being oxygenated.
39. The ____________ is a two-person device.
40. The most effective device for the PCT to use to ventilate the patient is the ____________.
41. Turn the pocket mask ____________ for infant resuscitation.
42. Insert an ____________ before using the bag-valve-mask device.
43. The ____________ must be fully stocked and ready to use at all times.
44. ____________ responds to defibrillation, whereas ____________ does not.
45. When the RN gives the command to defibrillate, you must ____________ quickly.
46. ____________ is care given to a patient who has been successfully resuscitated.
47. In health care facilities, the goal is to defibrillate within ____________ minutes.
48. Do not use the AED on a ____________.
49. After using the AED, crash cart, or other emergency equipment, you must ____________ supplies that were used.
50. A ____________ is a document that specifies the patient's wishes in the event of cardiac arrest.

Short Answer

Write the information in the space provided.

You are assigned to check the crash cart on the days listed during the month of July. Complete the crash cart checklist forms (pages 121 and 122) based on the information listed above each question.

July 1—Crash cart lock number D32579M, label OK, Ambu bag present with adult and pediatric masks, drug box lock number S893772K, drug box expired June 30, paper in defibrillator OK with spare roll present, defibrillator works at 200 joules, 6 packages Quik Combo patches present, oxygen cylinder has 750 pounds, 2 airways each size present, tape present, suction machine works, assorted flexible catheters present with 2 of each size, 2 Yankauers, curved blade light steady and white, straight blade light dim, one spare bulb present, 2 ET tubes of each size available, stylette present, no Kelly clamp.

51. What corrective action will you take? ______________________

____

July 2—Crash cart lock number D32579M, label OK, Ambu bag present with adult and pediatric masks, drug box lock number S893772K, drug box current, paper in defibrillator OK with spare roll present, defibrillator works at 200 joules, 6 packages Quik Combo patches present, oxygen cylinder has 750 pounds, 2 airways each size present, tape present, suction machine works, assorted flexible catheters present with 2 of each size, 2 Yankauers, curved blade light steady and white, straight blade light steady and white, no spare bulb present, 2 ET tubes of each size available, stylette present, Kelly clamp present.

52. What corrective action will you take? ______________________

____

July 3—Crash cart lock number P86631R, label OK, Ambu bag present with adult and pediatric masks, drug box lock number L321789D, drug box current, paper in defibrillator OK with spare roll present, defibrillator works at 200 joules, 4 packages Quik Combo patches present, oxygen cylinder has 450 pounds, 2 airways each size present, tape present, suction machine works, assorted flexible catheters present with 2 of each size, 2 Yankauers, curved blade light steady and white, straight blade light steady and white, spare bulb present, 2 ET tubes of each size available, stylette present, Kelly clamp present.

53. What corrective action will you take? ______________________

____

July 4—Crash cart lock number K75189T, label OK, Ambu bag present with adult and pediatric masks, drug box lock number S141680Z, drug box current, paper in defibrillator OK with spare roll present, defibrillator works at 200 joules, 3 packages Quik Combo patches present, oxygen cylinder has 825 pounds, 2 airways each size present, tape present, suction machine works, assorted flexible catheters present with 2 of each size, 1 Yankauer, curved blade light steady and white, straight blade light steady and white, spare bulb present, 2 ET tubes of each size available, stylette present, Kelly clamp present.

54. What corrective action will you take? ______________________

____

July 7—Crash cart lock number A34177R, label OK, Ambu bag present with adult and pediatric masks, drug box lock number P238641H, drug box current, paper in defibrillator OK with spare roll present, defibrillator works at 200 joules, 1 package Quik Combo patches present, oxygen cylinder has 525 pounds, 2 airways each size present, tape present, suction machine works, assorted flexible catheters present with 2 of each size, 3 Yankauers, curved blade light steady and white, straight blade light steady and white, spare bulb present, 2 ET tubes of each size available, stylette present, Kelly clamp present.

Crash Cart Checklist for July ______________, ______________

Month   Year

Signature/ Initials	Airways 2 each size	Tape (2)	Suction Working	Yankauer Caths (2)	Flexible Suction Caths-2 each size	Laryngoscope Light Works, Spare Bulb Present	Curved Blade (2)	Straight Blade (2)	ET Tubes-2 each size	Stylette & Kelly Clamp (1 each)

Crash Cart Checklist for ______July______, __________

Month Year

Date	Signature/ Initials	Crash Cart Lock #	Drug Box Lock #	500 PSI O_2 Cylinder Meter & Key in Place	Graph Paper in Defibrillator (plus 1-new roll)	Cart Label Current	If Expired, Cart Exchanged	Defibrillator Plugged In	Test at 200 Joules	Quik Combo Patches Present (6)	Ambu Bag Presen
1											
2											
3											
4											
5											
6											
7											
8											
9											
10											
11											
12											
13											
14											
15											
16											
17											
18											
19											
20											
21											
22											
23											
24											
25											
26											
27											
28											
29											
30											
31											

55. What corrective action will you take? ______________________________

____

July 11—Crash cart lock number B23160Y, label OK, Ambu bag present with adult and pediatric masks, drug box lock number J523698E, drug box current, paper in defibrillator OK with spare roll present, defibrillator works at 200 joules, 1 package Quik Combo patches present, oxygen cylinder has 900 pounds, 2 airways each size present, tape present, suction machine works, assorted flexible catheters present with 2 of each size, 2 Yankauers, curved blade light steady and white, straight blade light steady and white, spare bulb present, 2 ET tubes of each size available, stylette present, Kelly clamp present.

56. What corrective action will you take? ______________________________

____

July 14—Crash cart lock number Y90236U, label OK, Ambu bag present with adult masks, one pediatric mask missing, drug box lock number F150386M, drug box current, paper in defibrillator OK with spare roll present, defibrillator works at 200 joules, 6 packages Quik Combo patches present, oxygen cylinder has 850 pounds, 2 airways each size present, tape present, suction machine works, assorted flexible catheters present with 2 of each size, 2 Yankauers, curved blade light steady and white, straight blade light steady and white, spare bulb present, 2 ET tubes of each size available, no stylette, Kelly clamp present.

57. What corrective action will you take? ______________________________

____

July 19—Crash cart lock number Y31579N, label OK, Ambu bag present with adult and pediatric masks, drug box lock number W103226E, drug box current, paper in defibrillator OK, no spare roll available, defibrillator works at 200 joules, 5 packages Quik Combo patches present, oxygen cylinder has 750 pounds, 2 airways each size present, tape present, suction machine works, assorted flexible catheters present with 2 of each size, 2 Yankauers, curved blade light steady and white, straight blade light steady and white, spare bulb present, 2 ET tubes of each size available except size 7.0 has only one tube, stylette present, Kelly clamp present.

58. What corrective action will you take? ______________________________

____

July 24—Crash cart lock number A34177R, label OK, Ambu bag present with adult and pediatric masks, drug box lock number P238641H, drug box current, paper in defibrillator OK with spare roll present, defibrillator works at 200 joules, 6 packages Quik Combo patches present, oxygen cylinder has 750 pounds, 2 airways each size present, tape present, suction machine works, assorted flexible catheters present with 2 of each size, 2 Yankauers, curved blade light steady and white, straight blade light steady and white, spare bulb present, 2 ET tubes of each size available, stylette present, Kelly clamp present.

59. What corrective action will you take? ______________________________

____

July 30—Crash cart lock number R19875C, label OK, Ambu bag present with adult and pediatric masks, drug box lock number D196322V, drug box current, paper in defibrillator OK with spare roll present, defibrillator works at 200 joules, 4 packages Quik Combo patches present, oxygen cylinder has 950 pounds, 2 airways each size present, tape present, suction machine works, assorted flexible catheters present with 2 of each size, 2 Yankauers, curved blade light steady and white, straight blade light steady and white, spare bulb present, 2 ET tubes of each size available, stylette present, Kelly clamp present.

60. What corrective action will you take? ______________________________

____

Developing Greater Insight

Answer the following questions based on the situation described.

A 76-year-old female patient was transported to the emergency room by ambulance with complaints of chest pains and shortness of breath. The patient was placed in a room by herself. Staff did not continue the oxygen that had been administered in the ambulance. No one checked on the patient after she was placed in the room. A friend notified the family that the patient had been sent to the ER after complaining of chest pain at a church-sponsored bingo game. The patient's son and wife rushed to the hospital and were told that their mother was not there. Next, they went to the bingo hall, where they were told that their mother had been sent to the ER. They returned to the hospital, searched the ER, and found their mother in a room at the end of the hall. She was fully clothed with no oxygen or cardiac monitor. The son left the room to ask that someone come to help his mother. When he returned, the patient complained of indigestion. The son tried to help his mother to the bathroom, but she lost consciousness in the hallway. The son yelled for help. When personnel arrived, they called a code, but the patient could not be resuscitated. She was pronounced dead 1 hour and 15 minutes after the paramedics' record noted she had arrived at the hospital emergency room. There was a discrepancy between the time of arrival on the paramedic's run sheet and the ER record. The nurses altered the record.

61. If an ambulance brings a patient in with oxygen in use, how will you know whether to continue the oxygen?

____

____

62. How often should this patient's vital signs have been taken?

____

63. Should the patient have been connected to a cardiac monitor? Why or why not?

____

____

64. What action should be taken if there is a time discrepancy between the hospital record and the records of an external agency? ______________________________

____

65. The privacy laws make it difficult for staff to give out information as to whether a patient is receiving treatment. How will you know whether (when, and to whom) to give out information about whether a patient is present on your unit or emergency department? ______________________________

____

66. What signs and symptoms would you expect to see in a patient with chest pain who is in respiratory distress? ______________________________

____

The family sued the hospital for negligence and wrongful death. A jury found no liability on the part of the hospital. A lower court judge threw the verdict out in favor of undisclosed, but substantial, damages in favor of the family. The case went to the state court of appeals, which upheld the lower court judge's award of damages to the family. The appeals court did reduce the damages by 10 percent, because the judges believed there was a 90 percent likelihood that the patient would have survived the incident even without any negligence by the staff.

PART 2

Procedure and Student Performance Information

Beginning Procedure Actions

Procedure Completion Actions

Patient Care Technician Skill Checklist

Patient Care Technician Performance Record

Sample Patient Care Technician Performance Review Checklist

Patient Care Technician Performance Review Checklist

BEGINNING PROCEDURE ACTIONS

Beginning Procedure Action	Rationale
1. Wash your hands or use an alcohol-based hand cleaner.	Applies the principles of standard precautions. Prevents the spread of microbes and reduces the risk of cross-contamination.
2. Assemble equipment and take to the patient's room.	Improves efficiency of the procedure. Ensures that you do not have to leave the room.
3. Knock on the patient's door and identify yourself by name and title.	Respects the patient's right to privacy. Notifies the patient who is giving care.
4. Identify the patient by checking the identification bracelet.	Ensures that you are caring for the correct patient.
5. Ask visitors to leave the room and advise them where they may wait.	Respects the patient's right to privacy. Shows hospitality to visitors by advising them where to wait.
6. Explain what you are going to do and how the patient can assist. Answer questions about the procedure.	Informs the patient of what is going to be done and what is expected. Gives the patient an opportunity to get information about the procedure and the extent of patient participation.
7. Provide privacy by closing the door, privacy curtain, and window curtain.	Respects the patient's right to privacy. All three should be closed even if the patient is alone in the room.
8. Wash your hands or use an alcohol-based hand cleaner.	Applies the principles of standard precautions. Prevents the spread of microorganisms.
9. Set up the equipment for the procedure at the bedside. Open trays and packages. Position items in a location for convenient reach. Avoid positioning a container for soiled items in a manner that requires crossing over clean items to access it.	Prepares for the procedure. Ensures that the equipment and supplies are conveniently positioned and readily available. Reduces the risk of cross-contamination.
10. Raise the bed to a comfortable working height.	Prevents back strain and injury caused by bending at the waist.
11. Position the patient for the procedure. Ask an assistant to help, if necessary, or support the patient with pillows and props. Make sure the patient is comfortable and can maintain the position throughout the procedure. Drape the patient with a bath blanket for modesty.	Ensures that the patient is in the correct position for the procedure. Ensures that the patient is supported and can maintain the position without discomfort. Respects the patient's modesty and dignity.
12. Apply a gown if your uniform will have substantial contact with linen or other articles contaminated with blood, moist body fluid (except sweat), secretions, or excretions.	Applies the principles of standard precautions. Protects your uniform from contamination with bloodborne pathogens.
13. Apply a mask and eye protection if splashing of blood or moist body fluid is likely.	Applies the principles of standard precautions. Protects the PCT's mucous membranes, uniform, and skin from accidental splashing of bloodborne pathogens.
14. Apply gloves if contact with blood, moist body fluids (except sweat), secretions, excretions, or nonintact skin is likely.	Applies the principles of standard precautions. Protects the PCT and the patient from transmission of pathogens.
15. Lower the side rail on the side where you are working.	Provides an obstacle-free area in which to work.

PROCEDURE COMPLETION ACTIONS

Procedure Completion Actions	Rationale
1. Check to make sure the patient is comfortable and in good alignment.	All body systems function better when the body is correctly aligned. The patient is more comfortable when the body is in good alignment.
2. Remove gloves.	Prevents contamination of environmental surfaces from the gloves.
3. Replace the bed covers, then remove and discard any drapes used.	Provides warmth and security.
4. Elevate the side rails, if used, before leaving the bedside.	Prevents contamination of the side rail from used gloves. Supports the patient's right to a safe environment. Prevents accidents and injuries.
5. Remove other personal protective equipment, if worn, and discard according to facility policy.	Prevents unnecessary environmental contamination from used gloves and protective equipment.
6. Wash your hands, or use an alcohol-based hand cleaner.	Applies the principles of standard precautions. Prevents the spread of microorganisms.
7. Return the bed to the lowest horizontal position.	Supports the patient's right to a safe environment. Prevents accidents and injuries.
8. Open the privacy and window curtains.	Privacy is no longer necessary unless preferred by the patient.
9. Leave the patient in a position of comfort and safety with the call signal and needed personal items within reach.	Prevents accidents and injuries. Ensures that help is available. Eliminates the need to call or reach for needed personal items.
10. Wash your hands, or use an alcohol-based hand cleaner.	Although the hands were washed previously, they have contacted the patient and other items in the room. Wash them again before leaving to prevent potential transfer of microorganisms to areas outside the patient's unit.
11. Remove procedural trash and contaminated linen when you leave the room. Discard in appropriate container or location, according to facility policy.	Prevents the spread of microbes and reduces the risk of cross-contamination.
12. Inform visitors that they may return to the room.	Courtesy to visitors and the patient.
13. Report completion of the procedure and any abnormalities or other observations.	Informs the supervisor that your assigned task has been completed so further care can be planned and you can be reassigned to other duties. Notifies the licensed nurse of abnormalities and changes in the patient's condition that require further assessment.
14. Document the procedure and your observations.	Ongoing progress and care given are documented. Provides a legal record. Provides a record of what has been done for other members of the interdisciplinary team.

Patient Care Technician Skill Checklist

Instructions: This is a cumulative record of all the skills listed in your textbook, in numeric order. Have your instructor complete the record each time you have mastered a skill. Place the original in the permanent class file, and retain a copy for your records.

To the instructor: Feel free to duplicate the performance record. Fill in the skills that the student has completed. Retain the original in the master class file.

PATIENT CARE TECHNICIAN PERFORMANCE RECORD

Patient Care Technician Name (Last, First) ______________________

Social Security Number or ID Number ______________________

Program Name, Location ______________________

Dates of Class ____/____/____ to ____/____/____
mm dd yyyy mm dd yyyy

Program Code Number ______________________

S = Satisfactory Performance
U = Unsatisfactory Performance
* = See comments
Ints. = Initials

Place a full signature here to correspond with each set of initials on the form.

Initials	Corresponding Signature of Instructor	Title

NO. PROCEDURAL GUIDELINES	CLASSROOM			SKILLS LAB			CLINICAL		
	S/U	Date	Ints.	S/U	Date	Ints.	S/U	Date	Ints.
Chapter 3—Infection Control									
1. Handwashing									
2. Applying Disposable Gloves									
3. Removing Disposable Gloves									
4. Applying a Gown									
5. Removing a Gown									
6. Applying a Surgical Mask									
7. Removing a Surgical Mask									
8. Applying Protective Eyewear									
9. Removing Protective Eyewear									
10. Applying a NIOSH-Approved Respirator									
11. Removing a NIOSH-Approved Respirator									
Chapter 4—Surgical Asepsis									
12. Opening a Sterile Tray									
13. Opening a Sterile Package									
14. Setting Up a Sterile Field Using a Sterile Drape									
15. Adding an Item to a Sterile Field									
16. Adding Liquids to a Sterile Field									

(continues)

PATIENT CARE TECHNICIAN PERFORMANCE RECORD (CONTINUED)

NO. PROCEDURAL GUIDELINES	CLASSROOM			SKILLS LAB			CLINICAL		
	S/U	Date	Ints.	S/U	Date	Ints.	S/U	Date	Ints.
17. Applying and Removing Sterile Gloves									
18. Using Transfer Forceps									
Chapter 5—Wound Care									
19. Changing a Clean Dressing									
20. Applying a Bandage									
21. Applying a Sterile Dressing									
22. Applying a Dressing Around a Drain									
23. Changing Wet-to-Dry Dressings									
24. Applying a Transparent Film Dressing									
25. Applying a Hydrocolloid Dressing									
26. Pin Care									
27. Removing Sutures									
28. Removing Staples									
Chapter 6—Phlebotomy									
29. Performing a Venipuncture									
30. Collecting a Blood Specimen Using the Vacuum-Tube System									
31. Collecting a Blood Specimen Using a Butterfly Needle and Syringe									
32. Using the Blood Transfer Device									
33. Collecting a Blood Culture									
34. Drawing Blood Using a Lancet for a Microdraw or Infant Heel Stick									
35. Measuring Bleeding Time									
Chapter 7—Intravenous Therapy									
36. Assembling and Priming a Basic Administration Set									
37. Inserting a Peripheral IV in an Adult									
38. Inserting a Heparin Lock									

(continues)

PATIENT CARE TECHNICIAN PERFORMANCE RECORD (CONTINUED)

NO. PROCEDURAL GUIDELINES	CLASSROOM			SKILLS LAB			CLINICAL		
	S/U	Date	Ints.	S/U	Date	Ints.	S/U	Date	Ints.
39. Inserting an IV with a Butterfly Needle									
40. Inserting a Peripheral IV in a Child									
41. Monitoring the Intravenous Flow Rate									
42. Applying a Transparent Film Dressing to an Intravenous Infusion Site									
43. Discontinuing a Peripheral IV									
44. Assisting the RN with a Central IV Dressing Change									
45. Obtaining and Checking Blood from the Blood Bank									
46. Checking Blood Products on the Nursing Unit									
Chapter 8—Urinary and Bowel Elimination									
47. Testing Urine with Reagent Strips									
48. Measuring Urine Specific Gravity with a Urinometer									
49. Measuring Urine Specific Gravity with a Refractometer									
50. Multistix Urine Testing									
51. Inserting a Straight Catheter									
52. Inserting an Indwelling Catheter									
53. Changing a Nephrostomy Tube Dressing									
54. Open Bladder Irrigation									
55. Closed Bladder Irrigation									
56. Continuous Bladder Irrigation									
57. Removing an Indwelling Catheter									
58. Inserting a Rectal Tube and Flatus Bag									
59. Inserting a Rectal Suppository									
60. Administering a Cleansing Enema									
61. Administering a Commercially Prepared Enema									

(continues)

PATIENT CARE TECHNICIAN PERFORMANCE RECORD (CONTINUED)

NO. PROCEDURAL GUIDELINES	CLASSROOM			SKILLS LAB			CLINICAL		
	S/U	Date	Ints.	S/U	Date	Ints.	S/U	Date	Ints.
62. Breaking Up and Removing a Fecal Impaction									
63. Changing an Ostomy Appliance									
64. Irrigating a Colostomy									
Chapter 9—Enteral Nutrition									
65. Inserting a Nasogastric Tube									
66. Checking Nasogastric Tube Placement									
67. Aspirating for Residual Stomach Contents									
68. Irrigating a Nasogastric Tube									
69. Removing a Nasogastric Tube									
70. Gastrostomy Tube Care									
71. Inserting a Gastrostomy Tube into an Established Tract									
72. Bolus Enteral Feeding									
73. Continuous Enteral Feeding with a Pump									
Chapter 10—Specimen Collection									
74. Collecting a Throat Culture									
75. Obtaining a Swab Culture from a Wound									
76. Collecting a Sputum Specimen									
77. Collecting a Specimen for Gastric Analysis									
78. Collecting a Midstream Urine Sample									
79. Collecting a 24-Hour Urine Specimen									
80. Collecting a Sterile Urine Specimen from an Indwelling Catheter									
81. Obtaining a Urine Specimen Using the Speci-Cath Collection Device									
82. Straining the Urine for Renal Calculi									

(continues)

PATIENT CARE TECHNICIAN PERFORMANCE RECORD (CONTINUED)

NO. PROCEDURAL GUIDELINES	CLASSROOM			SKILLS LAB			CLINICAL		
	S/U	Date	Ints.	S/U	Date	Ints.	S/U	Date	Ints.
83. Collecting a Pediatric Urine Specimen									
84. Collecting a Stool Specimen									
85. Collecting a Rectal Swab Specimen for Culture and Sensitivity									
86. Collecting and Testing a Stool Specimen for Occult Blood									
87. Obtaining a Fingerstick Blood Sugar									
Chapter 11—Perioperative Care									
88. Shaving the Operative Site									
89. Coughing and Deep Breathing Exercises									
90. Incentive Spirometry									
91. Applying Antiembolism Stockings (Graduated Compression Hosiery)									
92. Applying the Pneumatic Compression Device									
93. Applying an Arm Sling									
94. Continuous Passive Motion Therapy									
95. Setting Up Traction (Claw-Type Basic Frame)									
Chapter 12—Heat and Cold Applications									
96. Applying a Hot Water Bottle, Gel Pack, or Chemical Hot Pack									
97. Performing a Warm Soak									
98. Applying Warm, Moist Compresses									
99. Applying an Aquathermia Pad (K-Pad)									
100. Applying Moist Hot Packs (Hydrocollator Tank)									
101. Giving a Tepid Sponge Bath to an Adult									
102. Giving a Tepid Bath to a Child									
103. Giving a Sitz Bath									

(continues)

PATIENT CARE TECHNICIAN PERFORMANCE RECORD (CONTINUED)

NO. PROCEDURAL GUIDELINES	CLASSROOM			SKILLS LAB			CLINICAL		
	S/U	Date	Ints.	S/U	Date	Ints.	S/U	Date	Ints.
104. Applying an Ice Bag, Ice Collar, Gel Pack, or Chemical Cold Pack									
105. Applying Cool, Moist Compresses									
106. Performing a Cool Soak									
107. Applying Warm or Cool Eye Compresses									
108. Applying the Hypothermia-Hyperthermia Blanket									
Chapter 13—Caring for Patients with Special Needs									
109. Caring for the Patient Who Is Having a Seizure									
Chapter 14—Respiratory Procedures									
110. Checking Capillary Refill									
111. Using a Pulse Oximeter									
112. Preparing Wall-Outlet Oxygen									
113. Preparing the Oxygen Cylinder									
114. Attaching the Humidifier to the Oxygen Flow Meter or Regulator									
115. Administering Oxygen Through a Nasal Cannula									
116. Administering Oxygen Through a Mask									
117. Inserting the Oropharyngeal Airway									
118. Inserting the Nasopharyngeal Airway									
119. Oropharyngeal Suctioning									
120. Nasopharyngeal Suctioning									
121. Administering a Small-Volume Nebulizer Treatment									
122. Assisting with Postural Drainage									
Chapter 15—Advanced Respiratory Procedures									
123. Assisting with Endotracheal Intubation									
124. Ventilating an Endotracheal Tube Using a Bag-Valve Device									

(continues)

PATIENT CARE TECHNICIAN PERFORMANCE RECORD (CONTINUED)

NO.	PROCEDURAL GUIDELINES	CLASSROOM			SKILLS LAB			CLINICAL		
		S/U	Date	Ints.	S/U	Date	Ints.	S/U	Date	Ints.
125.	Ventilating a Tracheostomy Using a Bag-Valve Device									
126.	Suctioning a Tracheostomy									
127.	Giving Tracheostomy/Stoma Care Using a Nondisposable Inner Cannula									
128.	Giving Tracheostomy/Stoma Care Using a Disposable Inner Cannula									
129.	Applying a Tracheostomy Dressing and Ties									
Chapter 16—Cardiac Care Skills										
130.	Performing a 12-Lead ECG									
131.	Setting Up for Continuous Cardiac Monitoring									
132.	Counting the Apical-Radial Pulse									
133.	Checking the Pulses in the Legs and Feet									
134.	Using a Dopper to Hear Pulse Sounds									
135.	Taking Blood Pressure with an Electronic Blood Pressure Apparatus									
136.	Monitoring after Cardiac Catheterization									
Chapter 17—Emergency Procedures										
137.	Head-Tilt, Chin-Lift Maneuver									
138.	Jaw-Thrust Maneuver									
139.	Obstructed Airway Procedure, Conscious Patient									
140.	Mouth-to-Mask Ventilation									
141.	Bag-Valve Mask Ventilation, Two Rescuers									
142.	One-Rescuer CPR, Adult									
143.	Two-Rescuer CPR, Adult									
144.	Positioning the Patient in the Recovery Position									

(continues)

PATIENT CARE TECHNICIAN PERFORMANCE RECORD (CONTINUED)

NO. PROCEDURAL GUIDELINES	CLASSROOM			SKILLS LAB			CLINICAL		
	S/U	Date	Ints.	S/U	Date	Ints.	S/U	Date	Ints.
145. Managing Cardiac Arrest Using an AED									
Appendix Procedures									
D1. Caring for a T-Tube or Similar Wound Drain									
D2. Caring for a Closed Wound Drainage System									
D3. Discontinuing an IV and Switching to a Heparin Lock									
D4. Applying a Holter Monitor									
List Facility and/or State-Specific Procedures Here									

(continues)

Comments (include date and signature/initials)

Patient Care Technician Performance Review Checklist

Instructions: This record lists the steps for each individual skill learned. List each step of the procedure numerically on a line, then complete the form. A completed example for the handwashing procedure is provided. Have your instructor complete the record each time you have mastered a skill. Place the original in the permanent class file, and retain a copy for your records.

Feel free to duplicate the blank performance review checklist. Fill in the skills the student has completed. Retain the original in the master class file.

SAMPLE PATIENT CARE TECHNICIAN PERFORMANCE REVIEW CHECKLIST

Patient Care Technician Name (Last, First) ____________________ Social Security Number or ID Number ____________________

Program Name, Location ____________________

Dates of Class ____/____/____ to ____/____/____
mm dd yyyy mm dd yyyy

Program Code Number ____________________

S = Satisfactory Performance
U = Unsatisfactory Performance
* = See comments
Ints. = Initials

Place a full signature here to correspond with each set of initials on the form.

Initials	Corresponding Signature of Instructor	Title

Procedure Number: 1
Procedure: HANDWASHING

PROCEDURAL GUIDELINES	S/U	Date	Initials	Comments
1. Turns on warm water.				
2. Wets hands. Keeps fingertips pointed down.				
3. Applies soap from dispenser.				
4. Rubs hands together vigorously to create a lather.				
• Rubs hands together in a circular motion for at least 15 seconds.				
• Rubs all surfaces of hands. Washes well between fingers.				
• Keeps fingertips pointed down.				
• Does not touch inside of sink or faucet handles.				
5. Rubs fingernails against palm of opposite hand. Cleans nails with brush or orange stick if soiled.				
6. Rinses hands from wrists to fingertips. Keeps fingers pointed down.				
7. Dries hands with a paper towel.				

(continues)

SAMPLE PATIENT CARE TECHNICIAN PERFORMANCE REVIEW CHECKLIST (CONTINUED)

PROCEDURAL GUIDELINES	S/U	Date	Initials	Comments
8. Uses clean, dry paper towel to turn off faucet.				
• Does not touch faucet handles with hands.				
9. Discards paper towel properly.				

Passed Skill ________ Failed Skill ________

________________________ ________________________
Instructor Signature Date

________________________ ________________________
Student Signature Date

PATIENT CARE TECHNICIAN PERFORMANCE REVIEW CHECKLIST

Patient Care Technician Name (Last, First) ______________________

Social Security Number or ID Number ______________________

Program Name, Location ______________________

Dates of Class ____/____/____ to ____/____/____
mm dd yyyy mm dd yyyy

Program Code Number ______________________

S = Satisfactory Performance
U = Unsatisfactory Performance
* = See comments
Ints. = Initials

Place a full signature here to correspond with each set of initials on the form.

Initials	Corresponding Signature of Instructor	Title

Procedure Number:
Procedure:

PROCEDURAL GUIDELINES	S/U	Date	Initials	Comments

Passed Skill __________ Failed Skill __________

____
Instructor Signature

____
Date

____
Student Signature

____
Date

PART 3

Documentation, Documentation Exercises, and Forms

Patient Care Technician Documentation: The Medical Record

Each health care facility must maintain clinical records on each patient, following accepted professional health information management standards. Documentation is the validation of quality care. Your instructor will stress that your job is not done until you have documented the care you have given.

All health status data about the patient must be available for all members of the health care team. The patient's medical records should be accessible, communicated, and recorded. Because all team members depend on the information in the medical record, documentation is a great responsibility. The record must be honest, objective, accurate, and complete. It must reflect the use of the nursing process, and show that the patient received care that met minimum acceptable standards. The American Nurses' Association (ANA) has made the following recommendations:

- ANA Standards of Clinical Nursing Practice should guide documentation
- Nurses should participate in designing documentation processes
- Documentation should promote "record once, read many times"
- ANA-recognized data sets should be utilized
- Nursing data must be retrievable, reusable, and able to support data analysis
- Professional nurses should critically evaluate documentation expectations

The adage "If it was not documented, it was not done" is as valid today as it was 50 years ago. In years past, some nurses viewed care as the main priority and treated documentation as secondary. Today, we cannot choose between giving care and keeping records. Both are important. In fact, the medical record and documentation *are part of* the patient's care, and validation of that care. Without accurate and complete documentation, no one knows with certainty what has been done. If the record is incomplete or inaccurate, it is difficult for caregivers to set goals or plan future clinical approaches for the patient's care.

Further, everyone who uses the records trusts that the data are accurate, honest, and objective. It is impossible for professionals to plan care to benefit the patient without accurate data. Accuracy means that the documentation reflects the care that was *actually* given, not the care that was *supposed to have been* given, but may or may not have been done. When the record is completely documented, it provides:

- The information needed to plan care
- The information needed to ensure continuity of care
- A means of communication between team members
- Written evidence of the rationale for treatments and care given
- Proof of modification of the care plan; the patient's response to the plan, and whether it was effective
- A means of monitoring patient care on an ongoing basis
- A vehicle for review, study, and evaluation of patient care

- A legal record that protects the patient, facility, and health care personnel
- A means of identifying and communicating information about the patient's problems, needs, and strengths

LEGAL EVIDENCE

Documentation is a legal record of each patient's care. As a legal document, the medical record can be used in a court of law. The notes are admitted as legal evidence. Lawyers, judges, juries, experts, and others may read them. If a medical record is used in a trial, the documentation shows that care was or was not given. This affects the outcome of the trial. When a note from the chart is used in a lawsuit, the worker who wrote the note may also have to testify at the trial. Testifying is a frightening, stressful experience. Lawsuits move very slowly through the courts. They often go to trial several years after care was given. You may not remember exactly what you did. Your notes must be complete and accurate, to prove what you did. Thorough notes help you defend your actions.

Your charting should leave no question in a reader's mind that you provided needed care and monitored the patient's condition. Tampering with, falsifying, altering, or destroying data in a patient's chart is illegal and unethical. One falsification can call the credibility of the entire record into question. By extension, the credibility and integrity of the personnel who documented in the record may also be questioned. Personnel may be charged with fraud based on falsification of records and documentation of care that was not provided. Charting in advance is also falsification. The only part of the record that may be documented in advance is the care plan. All other data are charted after being done.

Accountability

Everyone who cares for patients is responsible for documentation. Each worker is responsible for documenting the observations he or she makes and the services he or she provides. Health care workers *cannot* document for each other. Each worker is responsible for what he or she writes. Every entry in the chart is evidence that care was given. You cannot document care that you did not provide. For example, you know you must turn and reposition a patient every two hours. You will document that you turned the patient every two hours because you *actually did it,* not because that care was *supposed to have been given.*

Surveys

Surveyors review documentation when they visit the facility. Complete, accurate documentation proves that workers have complied with the law. It shows that patients have received good care. The record should show that patients' risks and needs were identified, and that care was given to meet them. Missing or absent documentation commonly results in deficiencies. Surveyors may ask questions about information in the chart. However, you should view documentation as something that helps care for the patient. It is much more than paper compliance!

DOCUMENTATION FORMAT

Many facilities use a system called *source-oriented medical records (SOMR).* The information in a SOMR is divided into categories. Each discipline has a separate divider in the chart in which the records for that discipline are stored. The sequence of the record varies from one facility to the next.

Some facilities use the *problem-oriented medical record (POMR).* This type of record is divided into five general categories, and all disciplines chart in each category. Facilities that use this system believe it improves communication. They state that it makes finding information easier.

Many different formats are used for recording information on the medical record. Medications, treatments, and ADLs are recorded on flow sheets. The caregiver initials a box, showing that care was given. Two other common formats are the narrative format and SOAP documentation. Facilities that use the *narrative format* describe the patient's care like a story. *SOAP* is an abbreviation for *Subjective, Objective, Assessment, Plan.* Facilities using this format write an entry for each category. For example:

- **S** stands for *subjective.* Because symptoms are subjective findings, they are described in this section. The patient, family member, or caregiver provides the information.
- **O** stands for *objective.* The information here is based on observations by the caregiver. The signs of the patient's condition are recorded here. Information about the patient's ability to function also goes in this section.
- **A** stands for *assessment.* The nurse practice act in most states prohibits unlicensed caregivers from cumulating the results of assessment data and formulating a plan of care. These things are the RN's responsibility. However, others may assist with assessments by collecting information, such as vital signs and other data. You report your findings to the RN. Because assessment is a professional responsibility, you must be careful about the wording of information written in this section. You may want to think of the "A" here as an abbreviation for *an analysis.* Because you are not legally permitted to assess, write your analysis of the situation here instead.
- **P** stands for *plan.* The plan describes the treatment information. You will document care listed in the plan for each patient.

Another popular system, similar to SOAP, is the *APIE system.* The meaning of this abbreviation is:

- **A** = assessment
- **P** = plan
- **I** = implementation of the plan
- **E** = evaluation of the patient's response to the plan.

Some facilities use a documentation system called *charting by exception* (*CBE*). In this system, normal findings and routine care are not documented. Only abnormals are documented. CBE is a formal system with policies, procedures, and special forms. It is not an informal method of documentation used because staff forgets to document. All nurse practice acts require nursing personnel to document care. Where, what form is used, and how this is done is up to the facility. A narrative note may not be necessary unless there is a deviation from normal. Exceptions to expected observations are always charted. Many facilities believe this is a risky method of charting, because it does not provide legal proof that care was given. Some facilities have had difficulty getting reimbursed for care without documentation to verify that it was given.

DOCUMENTING IN THE MEDICAL RECORD

Follow your facility policies and your state's legal guidelines for documentation. Most facilities use computers for documentation. Handwritten entries are not made unless the computer is not working (down). The facility will have a policy for using colored ink in the medical record. Chart only in the accepted color. Many facilities use only black, because it is clear and copies well. Avoid using erasable or nonpermanent ink. Remember that the medical record is a legal document that will be read by others. The information must always be accurate. Never record care you have not given. Avoid making up or overstating information.

Avoid providing the opportunity for the record to be altered. For example, notes written in pencil or erasable ink can be changed. Do not use these types of writing implements to document in medical records. Avoid leaving blank lines. These provide space for someone to change the record. If there are blank spaces, draw a line through them. This prevents others from filling them in. Never try to erase, obliterate, or white out an error. If you make an error, follow your facility policy for correcting it. In most facilities, you will draw a single line through the entry. Write the word "error" next to or above the entry. Sign the changes. Keep your documentation brief and concise.

Abbreviations

Use only acceptable, recognized abbreviations. Abbreviations are easily misunderstood, and some have more than one meaning. Limit your use of abbreviations and make sure the ones you do use are used correctly.

You will use some standard nursing abbreviations in your documentation. Many abbreviations are listed in your book. This was done so that you could understand documentation, and to provide a resource where you can check information you see in medical records and other documents in your facility. Your facility will have a specific list of abbreviations to use in charting. *Use only abbreviations that your facility accepts and recognizes.*

The JCAHO has approved a "minimum list" of dangerous abbreviations, acronyms, and symbols. These abbreviations may be misunderstood, and increase the risk of errors. Beginning January 1, 2004, accredited facilities must include certain items on their "do not use" lists. Of the abbreviations listed, the following are commonly used for PCT documentation:

- Q.D., Q.O.D. (Latin abbreviation for once daily and every other day)

The JCAHO requires facilities to periodically add other abbreviations to the "do not use" list. They recommend these for subsequent elimination from approved lists:

- H.S. (for half-strength or Latin abbreviation for bedtime)
- T.I.W. (for three times a week)
- D/C (for discharge)
- c.c. (for cubic centimeter)

The Institute for Safe Medication Practices has also updated its list of unsafe abbreviations. The ISMP recommends that the following be removed from use:

- OD (right eye)
- ʒ (dram)
- OJ (orange juice)
- per os (by mouth)
- qhs (nightly at bedtime)
- > < (greater than and less than)
- @ (at)
- & (and)
- + (plus or and)
- ° (hour)

Frequency of Documentation

A record is made each time you care for a patient. At the very least, you will initial a box on a flow sheet. You may be required to write a special note about an unusual situation, significant improvement, accident, or decline. Always document if the patient refuses treatment. If you are documenting a refusal on a flow sheet, place an "R" in the box. Explain the refusal on the back of the record or in a narrative note.

Timeliness of Documentation

Document your care in a timely manner. Never chart before providing care. Document as soon as possible after caring for the patient. Sometimes you cannot document immediately after caring for the patient. Carry a small notebook. Record important information that you can transfer to your notes later. If you forget to document something, then remember later, follow facility policy for late-entry documentation. Usually, you will write the date and time the entry is made. You will begin the entry by writing, "Late entry for (date, time)."

Understanding the Information

Your documentation must be clear to anyone who reads the chart. Your entries must be legible. Illegible information is easily misinterpreted. When documenting on flow sheets, make sure you use the correct box. If your handwriting is not legible, print. Your punctuation, grammar, and spelling must be correct. An accurate and concise record shows that you are conscientious. It implies that you have given quality care. Errors suggest that you are careless. If you are careless with your documentation, the reader may assume that you are careless with the care you give.

Signing the Entry

Follow your facility policy for signing each entry. Some facilities require you to sign your complete legal signature. Others use the first initial and last name. Your title and/or certification follow your name. Flow sheets will have a key for initials. Make sure you sign the key each month so others can identify your entries. Do not sign a flow sheet unless you are responsible for documenting on it. If you use a computerized documentation system, you will be permitted to use an electronic signature, but the facility will maintain an original copy of your signature. Your signature should always be legible.

Summary

As you can see, documentation is a key element of the care you give. It is not something you do strictly to satisfy regulations. Accurate, complete documentation benefits the patients and protects you legally. It ensures that the hospital or facility will be paid for the care provided. In turn, this enables the facility to meet payroll and pay its bills. Above all, it proves that you gave quality, conscientious care.

Documentation Exercises

CLINICAL SITUATION: CARING FOR MR. KOSMACEK

Mr. Henry Kosmacek was admitted to your rehabilitation unit on May 31 following an intensive care unit (ICU) stay for a stroke. He has left-side paralysis and is very weak. His speech is somewhat garbled. He has a history of congestive heart failure. He retains fluid when he is up, but puts out large amounts at night when he is in bed. His height is 68″, weight 146#, and vital signs 98.2°F (O) - 68 - 16 - 144/96. This 75-year-old widower has lived alone since his wife died 10 years ago. Before the stroke, he lived in a small house, and took great pleasure in tending his flower garden. He drove a car and went to the senior center daily. The doctor has ordered an intensive rehabilitation program. Mr. Kosmacek hopes to return home with a home health assistant.

Mr. Kosmacek can speak and make his needs known, but is forgetful. He uses a Foley catheter and is incontinent of stool. He has had trouble swallowing since the stroke, and an NG tube was inserted. He receives Glucerna bolus feedings every four hours. He wears glasses and hears normally. He needs assistance with bathing, dressing, and grooming. He has his own teeth, which are in good repair. His skin is dry and fragile, and tears easily. He is scheduled for a whirlpool bath on the day shift Monday, Wednesday, and Friday, and receives a bedbath on other days. He transfers with a transfer belt with one assistant. He needs a lap buddy when in the wheelchair to remind him not to get up alone. He has been unable to ambulate since the stroke, but can help by pivoting on his strong leg during transfers. The head of the bed must be elevated during feeding, and for an hour after feeding. The patient can turn to the left, but needs assistance turning to the right when in bed. His bed has four half rails. The two upper rails are pulled up to help the patient with turning. The ICU reports that he has never tried to get out of bed without help. The two lower side rails are down when he is in bed, and the nurse says they will evaluate his bed safety.

The nurse asked him about a numeric (1 to 10) pain scale, and he did not seem to understand the numbers. He seems to understand the Wong-Baker FACES pain scale, and admits to having chronic arthritic pain for which he receives a mild medication. The patient is frustrated because of his loss of independence.

Mr. Kosmacek has orders for TED hose when out of bed, PROM T.I.D., P.T. twice daily, an O.T. evaluation for self-help skills, speech evaluation for speaking and swallowing, and a nursing assessment for bowel and bladder retraining when the catheter is removed. The doctor has ordered intake and output monitoring, daily weight, and vital signs every four hours. The patient is not steady enough to use a standing scale, so you will use a chair or bed scale for measuring weight. The patient has an IV of 0.9 percent normal saline, and the nurse says this will be changed to a heparin lock soon. He has an order for fingerstick blood sugar readings every six hours, with sliding-scale insulin ordered. The RN schedules the FSBS for 11:30 p.m., 5:30 a.m., 11:30 a.m., and 5:30 p.m., so the insulin (if any) is given immediately before the tube feeding.

DOCUMENTATION ACTIVITIES

Ask your instructor to duplicate the forms in this section, if needed. Complete the documentation activities based on your knowledge of Mr. Kosmacek's history and physician orders (described in the preceding section) and the care (listed following). Use the forms in your workbook, or facility forms provided by your instructor.

ACTIVITY 1: Complete your admission documentation from your 9:00 a.m. admission data. The patient's height is 68″, weight 146#, and vital signs 98.2°F (O) - 68 - 16 - 144/96.

ACTIVITY 2: Mr. Kosmacek's IV infiltrated at 10:15 a.m. You restarted it in the left hand with a 22-gauge (long-dwell) needle. The patient is receiving 50 mL fluid per hour, and the nurse is running piggyback medications. Document your actions.

ACTIVITY 3: At 11:30 a.m., the FSBS is 264. You inform the RN. At 12:00 p.m., you take the patient's vital signs. They are 98.4°F (O) - 76 - 18 - 152/88. You check the tube feeding for residual and find 30 mL. You check the pH, which is 4.0, then return the fluid to the patient's stomach. You administer 300 mL Glucerna by bolus method of feeding in the NG tube, then flush the tube with 100 mL water as ordered. The head of the bed is elevated properly, and the patient tolerates the feeding well. Document your actions.

ACTIVITY 4: At the end of your shift, you must document intake and output. You have given Mr. Kosmacek 300 mL IV fluid, and 400 mL in the NG tube (300 mL Glucerna; 100 mL water). Nurses have written 240 mL additional fluid on the IV flow sheet during medication administration. There are 725 mL in the catheter bag. Document the I&O.

ACTIVITY 5: Monday, June 1—You are assigned to care for Mr. Kosmacek on the 7:00 a.m. to 3:00 p.m. shift. Select the correct forms and document the following care:

Vital signs, 8:00 a.m.: 97.4°F (O) - 64 - 16 - 126/88
Vital signs, 12:00 p.m.: 98.2°F (O) - 84 - 16 - 142/94
11:30 a.m. FSBS is 188. You inform the RN
Intake 800 mL in NG (600 mL Glucerna, 200 mL water), 360 mL medication water, 400 mL IV; output × 960 mL
Had a moderate BM (incontinent)
Bath: whirlpool with shampoo
Oral care: assist
Shave: self with electric razor and supervision
Nail care: nails cleaned
Linen change: complete
Activity: up in wheelchair with cushion to prevent skin breakdown, lap buddy used
Turned q2h in bed, repositioned q1h in w/c
Exercise: PROM × 2
Restraints: side rails × 2 in bed, lap buddy in chair
Bathing in whirlpool: self with one assist
Body alignment: self limited; one assist
Dressing: self with one assist
Toileting: Foley, catheter, and incontinent care given by staff
Grooming: self with one assist
Ambulation: dependent on staff, unable to propel wheelchair
Transfers: self with one assist

ACTIVITY 6: Tuesday, June 2—You are assigned to care for Mr. Kosmacek on the 7:00 a.m. to 3:00 p.m. shift. Select the correct forms and document the following care:

Vital signs, 8:00 a.m.: 97.2°F (O) - 60 - 16 - 132/86
Vital signs, 12:00 p.m.: 98.0°F (O) - 74 - 30 - 122/78
11:30 a.m. FSBS is 214. You inform the RN
Intake 800 mL in NG (600 mL Glucerna, 200 mL water), 360 mL medication water, 350 mL IV
Output × 720 mL
Foley catheter removed at 2:00 p.m. Has not voided since catheter removed
IV changed to heparin lock 2:00 p.m.
Moderate BM (incontinent)
Bath: BB
Oral care: assist
Shave: self with electric razor
Linen change: partial
Activity: up in wheelchair with cushion to prevent skin breakdown
Turned q2h in bed, repositioned q1h in w/c
Exercise: PROM × 2
Restraints: side rails × 2 in bed, lap buddy in chair
Bath: self with one assist
Body alignment: self limited; one assist
Dressing: self with one assist
Toileting: dependent on staff
Grooming: self with one assist
Ambulation: dependent on staff
Transfers: self with one assist

ACTIVITY 7: Wednesday, June 3—You are assigned to care for Mr. Kosmacek on the 6:00 a.m. to 2:00 p.m. shift. Complete the ADL sheet for your shift. Fill out a form with information you will turn in to the nurse at the end of the shift. Select the correct forms and document the following care:

Vital signs, 8:00 a.m.: 98.6°F (O) - 70 - 16 - 148/92
Vital signs, 12:00 p.m.: 99.2°F (O) - 80 - 20 - 154/86
11:30 a.m. FSBS is 132. You inform the RN
Intake 800 mL in NG (600 mL Glucerna, 200 mL water), 360 mL medication water
Output × incontinent of urine × 2
Large BM (incontinent)
B&B monitoring: 6:00 a.m. dry, 7:00 a.m. dry, 8:00 a.m. dry, 9:00 a.m. incontinent large urine and BM, 10:00 a.m. dry, 11:00 a.m. dry, 12:00 p.m. dry, 1:00 p.m. incontinent large, 2:00 p.m. dry
Bath: whirlpool with shampoo
Oral care: assist
Shave: self with electric razor
Nail care: nails cleaned
Linen change: complete
Activity: up in wheelchair with cushion to prevent skin breakdown
Turned q2h in bed, repositioned q1h in w/c

Exercise: PROM × 2
Restraints: side rails × 2 in bed, lap buddy in chair
Bathing in whirlpool: self with one assist
Body alignment: self limited; one assist
Dressing: self with one assist
Toileting: dependent on staff
Grooming: self with one assist
Ambulation: dependent on staff
Transfers: self with one assist

ACTIVITY 8: Thursday, June 4—You are assigned to care for Mr. Kosmacek on the 6:00 a.m. to 2:00 p.m. shift. Complete the ADL sheet for your shift. Fill out a form with information you will turn in to the nurse at the end of the shift. Select the correct forms and document the following care:

Vital signs, 8:00 a.m.: 98.4°F (O) - 76 - 18 - 136/76
Vital signs, 12:00 p.m.: 97.8°F (O) - 74 - 14 - 140/82
11:30 a.m. FSBS is 306. You inform the RN
Intake 800 mL in NG (600 mL Glucerna, 200 mL water), 360 mL medication water
Output = incontinent × 4
No BM
B&B monitoring: 6:00 a.m. wet large, 7:00 a.m. dry, 8:00 a.m. wet small, 9:00 a.m. dry, 10:00 a.m. dry, 11:00 a.m. wet moderate, 12:00 p.m. dry, 1:00 p.m. dry, 2:00 p.m. wet large
Bath: whirlpool with shampoo
Oral care: assist
Shave: self with electric razor
Linen change: complete
Activity: up in wheelchair with cushion to prevent skin breakdown
Turned q2h in bed, repositioned q1h in w/c
Exercise: PROM × 2
Restraints: side rails × 2 in bed, lap buddy in chair
Bedbath: self with one assist
Body alignment: self limited; one assist
Dressing: self with one assist
Toileting: dependent on staff
Grooming: self with one assist
Ambulation: dependent on staff
Transfers: self with one assist

ACTIVITY 9: Monday, June 8—You are assigned to care for Mr. Kosmacek on the 7:00 a.m. to 3:00 p.m. shift. Complete the ADL sheet for your shift. Select the correct forms and document the following care:

Vital signs, 8:00 a.m.: 98°F (O) - 80 - 20 - 146/88
Vital signs, 12:00 p.m.: 97.4°F (O) - 68 - 14 - 126/94
11:30 a.m. FSBS is 164. You inform the RN
Weight: 140
Intake 800 mL in NG (600 mL Glucerna, 200 mL water), 360 mL medication water
Output = incontinent × 3

Had a moderate BM (incontinent)

B&B monitoring: 6:00 a.m. dry, 7:00 a.m. wet large, 8:00 a.m. dry, 9:00 a.m. dry, 10:00 a.m. wet large urine, incontinent mod BM, 11:00 a.m. dry, 12:00 p.m. dry, 1:00 p.m. wet small, 2:00 p.m. dry

Bath: whirlpool with shampoo

Oral care: assist

Shave: self with electric razor

Nail care: nails cleaned

Linen change: partial

Activity: up in wheelchair with cushion to prevent skin breakdown

Turned q2h in bed, repositioned q1h in w/c

Exercise: PROM × 2

Restraints: side rails × 2 in bed, lap buddy in chair

The dietitian evaluated the patient and noted he was at the low end of his ideal body weight range of 139 to 169 pounds. She recommended increasing the caloric intake from 1,800 calories daily to 2,200 calories. The nurse has put in a call to the physician and is awaiting a return call.

FORMS FOR DOCUMENTATION ACTIVITIES

ADL FLOWSHEET

	HR	1	2	3	4	5	6	7	8	9	10	11	12	13	14	15	16	17	18	19	20	21	22	23	24	25	26	27	28	29	30	31
DIET: 75% (GOOD) 50% (FAIR) 25% (POOR) S + SUBSTITUTE ( ) DINING ROOM ( ) FEEDS SELF	B																															
	L																															
	D																															
	S																															
Bath ( ) Bed Bath (BB) ( ) Whirlpool (WP) ( ) Shower (S) ( ) Tub Bath (TB) ( ) Partial Bath (PB) ( ) Independent (I) ( ) Assistance (A) ( ) Total Help (TH)	D																															
	E																															
Oral Care ( ) Dentures ( ) Own Teeth ( ) Special Instructions ( ) Independent (I) ( ) Assistance (A) ( ) Total Help (TH)	N																															
	D																															
	E																															
Fingernail Care ( ) Independent (I) ( ) Assist (A) ( )Total Help (TH) Toenail Care ( ) Independent (I) ( ) Assist (A) ( )Total Help (TH)	N																															
	N																															
Shave ( ) Independent (I) ( ) Assist (A) ( )Total Help (TH) Shampoo ( ) Independent (I) ( ) Assist (A) ( )Total Help (TH)	S																															
	S																															
Bowel Movement (BM) L = Large M = Medium S = Small	N																															
	D																															
	E																															
( ) Incontinent (I) ( ) Continent (C) ( ) Urine ( ) Incontinent (I) ( ) Continent (C) ( ) Feces ( ) Partial bath/Peri-Care after each incontinent episode	N																															
	D																															
	E																															
Skin Care ( ) Turn and reposition Q2h ( ) Peri-Care ( ) Backrub ( ) Other: ______	N																															
	D																															
	E																															
Ambulation ( ) Ambulatory (I) ( ) Partial Bedfast ( ) Walker ( ) Geri-chair ( ) Cane ( ) Wheelchair ( ) Independent (I) ( ) Assist (A) ( ) Total Help (TH)	N																															
	D																															
	E																															
Protective Safety Device Q 1 hour, R/R Q 2 hours × 10 min. ( ) Vest ( ) Side Rails: ____ ( ) Waist ( ) Geri-chair ( ) Lap Buddy ( ) Other: ______	N																															
	D																															
	E																															
Routine Resident Check Q 2 hours ( ) Offered Fluids Q 2 hours ( )	N																															
	D																															
	E																															
Linen Change Total (T) Partial (P)	N																															
	D																															
	E																															

Indicate Temp. in Black and Pulse in Red Ink

DATE / HOSP. DAY							
POST-OP. DAY							
PULSE / F.	4 8 12 4 8 12	4 8 12 4 8 12	4 8 12 4 8 12	4 8 12 4 8 12	4 8 12 4 8 12	4 8 12 4 8 12	4 8 12 4 8 12
150 / 106°							
140 / 105°							
130 / 104°							
120 / 103°							
110 / 102°							
100 / 101°							
90 / 100°							
80 / 99°							
70 / 98°							
60 / 97°							
50 / 96°							
40 / 95°							
Resp. Rate							
Blood Pressure	7-3 3-11 11-7	7-3 3-11 11-7	7-3 3-11 11-7	7-3 3-11 11-7	7-3 3-11 11-7	7-3 3-11 11-7	7-3 3-11 11-7
Fluid Intake-Oral							
Parenteral							
Blood Transfusion							
24-Hr. Intake Total							
Fluid Output-Urine							
Gastric Suction							
Emesis							
Other							
24-Hr. Output Total							
Stool							
Height/Weight							
FSBS (fingerstick bloodsugar)	7 11 4 9	7 11 4 9	7 11 4 9	7 11 4 9	7 11 4 9	7 11 4 9	7 11 4 9
Acetest							

IMPRINT AREA

GRAPHIC RECORD

DATE																																				
HOSPITAL DAY																																				
POST-OP DAY																																				
TIME	12	4	8	12	4	8	12	4	8	12	4	8	12	4	8	12	4	8	12	4	8	12	4	8	12	4	8	12	4	8	12	4	8	12	4	8
TEMPERATURE																																				
105°																																				
104°																																				
103°																																				
102°																																				
101°																																				
100°																																				
99°																																				
98°																																				
97°																																				
PULSE																																				
170																																				
160																																				
150																																				
140																																				
130																																				
120																																				
110																																				
100																																				
90																																				
80																																				
RESPIRATION																																				
70																																				
60																																				
50																																				
40																																				
30																																				
20																																				
10																																				
BLOOD PRESSURE AM	12		4		8		12		4		8		12		4		8		12		4		8		12		4		8		12		4		8	
BLOOD PRESSURE PM	12		4		8		12		4		8		12		4		8		12		4		8		12		4		8		12		4		8	
WEIGHT / STOOL																																				

INTAKE-OUTPUT WORKSHEET

Intake Equivalents

Medicine Cup - 30 mL	Soup Bowl 8 oz/240 mL	Water Pitcher - 1,000 mL
Water Glass 8 oz - 240 mL	Styrofoam Cup 6 oz/180 mL	Juice Glass 4 oz/120 mL
Ice Cream 3 oz - 90 mL	Carton Milk 8 oz/240 mL	Coffee Cup 6 oz/180 mL

Time	Intake	Output	
	NOC	URINE	EMESIS
			BM
			DRAINAGE

Time	Intake	Output	
	AM	URINE	EMESIS
			BM
			DRAINAGE

Time	Intake	Output	
	PM	URINE	EMESIS
			BM
			DRAINAGE

Measurements are guidelines only. Verify container size used in your facility.

PATIENT: ______________________________

ROOM: ______________________________

DATE: ______________________________

INTAKE & OUTPUT SUMMARY

Month ________________ Year ________

DATE	SHIFT	INTAKE	OUTPUT	DATE	SHIFT	INTAKE	OUTPUT	DATE	SHIFT	INTAKE	OUTPUT	DATE	SHIFT	INTAKE	OUTPUT
1	NOC			2	NOC			3	NOC			4	NOC		
	AM				AM				AM				AM		
	PM				PM				PM				PM		
*	24 HR. TOTAL			*	24 HR. TOTAL			*	24 HR. TOTAL			*	24 HR. TOTAL		
5	NOC			6	NOC			7	NOC			8	NOC		
	AM				AM				AM				AM		
	PM				PM				PM				PM		
*	24 HR. TOTAL			*	24 HR. TOTAL			*	24 HR. TOTAL			*	24 HR. TOTAL		
9	NOC			10	NOC			11	NOC			12	NOC		
	AM				AM				AM				AM		
	PM				PM				PM				PM		
*	24 HR. TOTAL			*	24 HR. TOTAL			*	24 HR. TOTAL			*	24 HR. TOTAL		
13	NOC			14	NOC			15	NOC			16	NOC		
	AM				AM				AM				AM		
	PM				PM				PM				PM		
*	24 HR. TOTAL			*	24 HR. TOTAL			*	24 HR. TOTAL			*	24 HR. TOTAL		

*Document in N/N inadequate 24hour I&O's–Note color, odor, Nrsg intervention, etc.

PATIENT NAME ________________ PHYSICIAN ________________ ROOM NO. ________

INTAKE & OUTPUT SUMMARY

Month ________________ Year ______

DATE	SHIFT	INTAKE	OUTPUT	DATE	SHIFT	INTAKE	OUTPUT	DATE	SHIFT	INTAKE	OUTPUT	DATE	SHIFT	INTAKE	OUTPUT
17	NOC			18	NOC			19	NOC			20	NOC		
	AM				AM				AM				AM		
	PM				PM				PM				PM		
*	24 HR. TOTAL			*	24 HR. TOTAL			*	24 HR. TOTAL			*	24 HR. TOTAL		
21	NOC			22	NOC			23	NOC			24	NOC		
	AM				AM				AM				AM		
	PM				PM				PM				PM		
*	24 HR. TOTAL			*	24 HR. TOTAL			*	24 HR. TOTAL			*	24 HR. TOTAL		
25	NOC			26	NOC			27	NOC			28	NOC		
	AM				AM				AM				AM		
	PM				PM				PM				PM		
*	24 HR. TOTAL			*	24 HR. TOTAL			*	24 HR. TOTAL			*	24 HR. TOTAL		
29	NOC			30	NOC			31	NOC						
	AM				AM				AM						
	PM				PM				PM						
*	24 HR. TOTAL			*	24 HR. TOTAL			*	24 HR. TOTAL						

*Document in N/N inadequate 24hour I&O's–Note color, odor, Nrsg intervention, etc.

PATIENT NAME ______________________ PHYSICIAN ______________________ ROOM NO. __________

DAILY INTAKE AND OUTPUT

DATE:

PARENTERAL	HR.	I.V.	ORAL	CBI	TOTAL URINE	TRUE URINE	OTHER CATH.	STOOL	GASTRIC	EMESIS	DRAIN
CT:	2400										
	100										
	200										
	300										
11-7	400										
	500										
	600										
	700										
Total 8 Hrs.											
CT:	800										
	900										
	1000										
	1100										
7-3	1200										
	1300										
	1400										
	1500										
Total 8 Hrs.											
CT:	1600										
	1700										
	1800										
	1900										
3-11	2000										
	2100										
	2200										
	2300										
Total 8 Hrs.											
Total 24 Hrs.											

INITIAL INCONTINENCE EVALUATION (VOIDING PATTERN ASSESSMENT)

○ ○ ∅ — Incontinent SMALL AMOUNT
○ ∅ ○ — Incontinent MODERATE AMOUNT
∅ ○ ○ — Incontinent LARGE AMOUNT

• Dry when checked
(/) Stool present
(X) Resident asked to use toilet

Day ______________________ Date _____/_____/_____

NURSING ASSISTANT	TIME	INCONTINENT	DRY	STOOL	PATIENT REQUESTED	TOILETED
	12 MIDNIGHT	○ ○ ○	●	( )	( )	mL
	1 AM	○ ○ ○	●	( )	( )	mL
	2 AM	○ ○ ○	●	( )	( )	mL
	3 AM	○ ○ ○	●	( )	( )	mL
	4 AM	○ ○ ○	●	( )	( )	mL
	5 AM	○ ○ ○	●	( )	( )	mL
	6 AM	○ ○ ○	●	( )	( )	mL
	7 AM	○ ○ ○	●	( )	( )	mL
	8 AM	○ ○ ○	●	( )	( )	mL
	9 AM	○ ○ ○	●	( )	( )	mL
	10 AM	○ ○ ○	●	( )	( )	mL
	11 AM	○ ○ ○	●	( )	( )	mL
	12 PM	○ ○ ○	●	( )	( )	mL
	1 PM	○ ○ ○	●	( )	( )	mL
	2 PM	○ ○ ○	●	( )	( )	mL
	3 PM	○ ○ ○	●	( )	( )	mL
	4 PM	○ ○ ○	●	( )	( )	mL
	5 PM	○ ○ ○	●	( )	( )	mL
	6 PM	○ ○ ○	●	( )	( )	mL
	7 PM	○ ○ ○	●	( )	( )	mL
	8 PM	○ ○ ○	●	( )	( )	mL
	9 PM	○ ○ ○	●	( )	( )	mL
	10 PM	○ ○ ○	●	( )	( )	mL
	11 PM	○ ○ ○	●	( )	( )	mL
TOTALS						mL

PATIENT NAME: ________________________________ ROOM NO. ____________

I.V. FLOW SHEET

INITIATION

DATE/TIME	SITE	TYPE/SIZE CATH.	INITIAL

DISCONTINUED

DATE/TIME	REASON	INITIAL	SITE STATUS	TUBING CHANGE	INITIAL

REASON START/RESTART:
A. New I.V.
B. Painful
C. Erythema
D. Induration
E. Infiltration
F. Other
G. Occlusion
H. 72 Hour
I. Pulled out
J. Physician's orders

SITE:
A. Hand Metacarpal
B. Dorsal Forearm
C. Ventral Forearm
D. Antecubital
E. Upper Arm
F. Wrist
G. Jugular
H. Subclavian
I. Feet
J. Other

SITE STATUS:
A. Without Erythema, Pain
B. Painful
C. Erythema
D. Induration
E. Infiltration
F. Other

PARENTERAL FLUID RECORD

DATE/TIME	SITE	SOLUTION	RATE	MEDICATION	SIGNATURE	TIME D/Cd	AMT. INFUSED	IN ORAL	OUT	SIGNATURE

LAST NAME FIRST NAME ATTENDING PHYSICIAN ROOM NO.

TUBE FEEDING RECORD

TUBE FEEDING ORDER: ______________________________

DATE	SHIFT	FORMULA INTAKE ml's	PHYSICIAN ORDERED WATER INTAKE	IRRIGATION/ FLUSH H_2O INTAKE	MED. ADM. WATER INTAKE	ORAL FLUID INTAKE	TOTAL FLUID INTAKE	TOTAL OUTPUT (ml's or # of X's)

PATIENT: ______________________________ ROOM NO.: ______________

PHYSICIAN: ______________________________

TUBE FEEDING RECORD

FORMULA ___	HR	1	2	3	4	5	6	7	8	9	10	11	12	13	14	15	16	17	18	19	20	21	22	23	24	25	26	27	28	29	30	31
at ___ mL/ ___ HR via	HR	1	2	3	4	5	6	7	8	9	10	11	12	13	14	15	16	17	18	19	20	21	22	23	24	25	26	27	28	29	30	31
GRAVITY ☐ PUMP ☐ BOLUS ☐	HR	1	2	3	4	5	6	7	8	9	10	11	12	13	14	15	16	17	18	19	20	21	22	23	24	25	26	27	28	29	30	31
TOTAL CALORIES PER 24 HRS. ___	HR	1	2	3	4	5	6	7	8	9	10	11	12	13	14	15	16	17	18	19	20	21	22	23	24	25	26	27	28	29	30	31
	HR	1	2	3	4	5	6	7	8	9	10	11	12	13	14	15	16	17	18	19	20	21	22	23	24	25	26	27	28	29	30	31
	HR	1	2	3	4	5	6	7	8	9	10	11	12	13	14	15	16	17	18	19	20	21	22	23	24	25	26	27	28	29	30	31
	HR	1	2	3	4	5	6	7	8	9	10	11	12	13	14	15	16	17	18	19	20	21	22	23	24	25	26	27	28	29	30	31
	HR	1	2	3	4	5	6	7	8	9	10	11	12	13	14	15	16	17	18	19	20	21	22	23	24	25	26	27	28	29	30	31
CHECK TUBE PLACEMENT PRIOR TO	HR	1	2	3	4	5	6	7	8	9	10	11	12	13	14	15	16	17	18	19	20	21	22	23	24	25	26	27	28	29	30	31
EACH FEEDING OR MEDICATION	HR	1	2	3	4	5	6	7	8	9	10	11	12	13	14	15	16	17	18	19	20	21	22	23	24	25	26	27	28	29	30	31
ADMINISTRATION BY AIR	HR	1	2	3	4	5	6	7	8	9	10	11	12	13	14	15	16	17	18	19	20	21	22	23	24	25	26	27	28	29	30	31
AUSCULTATION/ASPIRATION	HR	1	2	3	4	5	6	7	8	9	10	11	12	13	14	15	16	17	18	19	20	21	22	23	24	25	26	27	28	29	30	31
	HR	1	2	3	4	5	6	7	8	9	10	11	12	13	14	15	16	17	18	19	20	21	22	23	24	25	26	27	28	29	30	31
CHECK TUBE RESIDUAL. IF OVER ___ mL	HR	1	2	3	4	5	6	7	8	9	10	11	12	13	14	15	16	17	18	19	20	21	22	23	24	25	26	27	28	29	30	31
HOLD FEEDING & NOTIFY DOCTOR. RETURN	HR	1	2	3	4	5	6	7	8	9	10	11	12	13	14	15	16	17	18	19	20	21	22	23	24	25	26	27	28	29	30	31
CONTENTS TO STOMACH 1 x PER SHIFT.	HR	1	2	3	4	5	6	7	8	9	10	11	12	13	14	15	16	17	18	19	20	21	22	23	24	25	26	27	28	29	30	31
ORAL & NARES HYGIENE	HR	1	2	3	4	5	6	7	8	9	10	11	12	13	14	15	16	17	18	19	20	21	22	23	24	25	26	27	28	29	30	31
Q SHIFT & PRN	HR	1	2	3	4	5	6	7	8	9	10	11	12	13	14	15	16	17	18	19	20	21	22	23	24	25	26	27	28	29	30	31
	HR	1	2	3	4	5	6	7	8	9	10	11	12	13	14	15	16	17	18	19	20	21	22	23	24	25	26	27	28	29	30	31
	HR	1	2	3	4	5	6	7	8	9	10	11	12	13	14	15	16	17	18	19	20	21	22	23	24	25	26	27	28	29	30	31
PUMP IS FREE OF DUST, DIRT, RESIDUE	HR	1	2	3	4	5	6	7	8	9	10	11	12	13	14	15	16	17	18	19	20	21	22	23	24	25	26	27	28	29	30	31
Q SHIFT. CLEAN PUMP Q DAY.	HR	1	2	3	4	5	6	7	8	9	10	11	12	13	14	15	16	17	18	19	20	21	22	23	24	25	26	27	28	29	30	31
	HR	1	2	3	4	5	6	7	8	9	10	11	12	13	14	15	16	17	18	19	20	21	22	23	24	25	26	27	28	29	30	31
	HR	1	2	3	4	5	6	7	8	9	10	11	12	13	14	15	16	17	18	19	20	21	22	23	24	25	26	27	28	29	30	31
VISUAL CHECK OF TUBE	HR	1	2	3	4	5	6	7	8	9	10	11	12	13	14	15	16	17	18	19	20	21	22	23	24	25	26	27	28	29	30	31
PLACEMENT Q 1 HOUR.	HR	1	2	3	4	5	6	7	8	9	10	11	12	13	14	15	16	17	18	19	20	21	22	23	24	25	26	27	28	29	30	31
	HR	1	2	3	4	5	6	7	8	9	10	11	12	13	14	15	16	17	18	19	20	21	22	23	24	25	26	27	28	29	30	31
	HR	1	2	3	4	5	6	7	8	9	10	11	12	13	14	15	16	17	18	19	20	21	22	23	24	25	26	27	28	29	30	31
CHANGE NGT Q MONTH USING	HR	1	2	3	4	5	6	7	8	9	10	11	12	13	14	15	16	17	18	19	20	21	22	23	24	25	26	27	28	29	30	31
	HR	1	2	3	4	5	6	7	8	9	10	11	12	13	14	15	16	17	18	19	20	21	22	23	24	25	26	27	28	29	30	31
FR # ___	HR	1	2	3	4	5	6	7	8	9	10	11	12	13	14	15	16	17	18	19	20	21	22	23	24	25	26	27	28	29	30	31
	HR	1	2	3	4	5	6	7	8	9	10	11	12	13	14	15	16	17	18	19	20	21	22	23	24	25	26	27	28	29	30	31
MAY REINSERT NGT PRN PATENCY POSITION	HR	1	2	3	4	5	6	7	8	9	10	11	12	13	14	15	16	17	18	19	20	21	22	23	24	25	26	27	28	29	30	31
	HR	1	2	3	4	5	6	7	8	9	10	11	12	13	14	15	16	17	18	19	20	21	22	23	24	25	26	27	28	29	30	31
USING FR # ___	HR	1	2	3	4	5	6	7	8	9	10	11	12	13	14	15	16	17	18	19	20	21	22	23	24	25	26	27	28	29	30	31
	HR	1	2	3	4	5	6	7	8	9	10	11	12	13	14	15	16	17	18	19	20	21	22	23	24	25	26	27	28	29	30	31
CHANGE FEEDING BAG AND	HR	1	2	3	4	5	6	7	8	9	10	11	12	13	14	15	16	17	18	19	20	21	22	23	24	25	26	27	28	29	30	31
TUBING Q 24 HRS.	HR	1	2	3	4	5	6	7	8	9	10	11	12	13	14	15	16	17	18	19	20	21	22	23	24	25	26	27	28	29	30	31
	HR	1	2	3	4	5	6	7	8	9	10	11	12	13	14	15	16	17	18	19	20	21	22	23	24	25	26	27	28	29	30	31
	HR	1	2	3	4	5	6	7	8	9	10	11	12	13	14	15	16	17	18	19	20	21	22	23	24	25	26	27	28	29	30	31
HOB ELEVATED 30' OR MORE	HR	1	2	3	4	5	6	7	8	9	10	11	12	13	14	15	16	17	18	19	20	21	22	23	24	25	26	27	28	29	30	31
AT ALL TIMES.	HR	1	2	3	4	5	6	7	8	9	10	11	12	13	14	15	16	17	18	19	20	21	22	23	24	25	26	27	28	29	30	31
	HR	1	2	3	4	5	6	7	8	9	10	11	12	13	14	15	16	17	18	19	20	21	22	23	24	25	26	27	28	29	30	31
	HR	1	2	3	4	5	6	7	8	9	10	11	12	13	14	15	16	17	18	19	20	21	22	23	24	25	26	27	28	29	30	31
	HR	1	2	3	4	5	6	7	8	9	10	11	12	13	14	15	16	17	18	19	20	21	22	23	24	25	26	27	28	29	30	31
FLUSH TUBE WITH ___ mL WATER	HR	1	2	3	4	5	6	7	8	9	10	11	12	13	14	15	16	17	18	19	20	21	22	23	24	25	26	27	28	29	30	31
BEFORE / AFTER MEDICATIONS &	HR	1	2	3	4	5	6	7	8	9	10	11	12	13	14	15	16	17	18	19	20	21	22	23	24	25	26	27	28	29	30	31
Q TIME FEEDING IS STOPPED / STARTED	HR	1	2	3	4	5	6	7	8	9	10	11	12	13	14	15	16	17	18	19	20	21	22	23	24	25	26	27	28	29	30	31
FLUSH TUBE WITH ___ mL WATER	HR	1	2	3	4	5	6	7	8	9	10	11	12	13	14	15	16	17	18	19	20	21	22	23	24	25	26	27	28	29	30	31
	HR	1	2	3	4	5	6	7	8	9	10	11	12	13	14	15	16	17	18	19	20	21	22	23	24	25	26	27	28	29	30	31
	HR	1	2	3	4	5	6	7	8	9	10	11	12	13	14	15	16	17	18	19	20	21	22	23	24	25	26	27	28	29	30	31
Q SHIFT TO TOTAL ___ mL/24 HRS.	HR	1	2	3	4	5	6	7	8	9	10	11	12	13	14	15	16	17	18	19	20	21	22	23	24	25	26	27	28	29	30	31

PATIENT ___

MONTH/YEAR ___

ROOM # ___

INITIALS	SIGNATURE
INITIALS	SIGNATURE
INITIALS	SIGNATURE
INITIALS	SIGNATURE

FINGER STICK / BLOOD SUGAR RECORD

		1	2	3	4	5	6	7	8	9	10	11	12	13	14	15	16	17	18	19	20	21	22	23	24	25	26	27	28	29	30	31
PLACE ACTUAL FINGER STICK ORDER IN THIS BOX — TIMES	HR																															
	HR																															
	HR																															
	HR																															
	HR																															
	HR																															
NOTIFY PHYSICIAN IF FS↓ ________ or ↑ ________ — TIMES	HR																															
	HR																															
	HR																															
	HR																															
	HR																															
	HR																															
READING																																
READING																																
READING																																
READING																																
READING																																
READING																																
READING																																

PATIENT ________________________

MONTH/YEAR ________________________

ROOM # ________________________

INITIALS	SIGNATURE
INITIALS	SIGNATURE
INITIALS	SIGNATURE
INITIALS	SIGNATURE

DATE	TIME	NURSE'S NOTES

PATIENT'S NAME PHYSICIAN ROOM #